THE TOP 100
HEALTH
TIPS

THE TOP 100 HEALTH TIPS

JANET WRIGHT

DUNCAN BAIRD PUBLISHERS

LONDON

To my mother Marie Joan Wright and to my husband David Hall

THE TOP 100 HEALTH TIPS
Janet Wright

First published in the United Kingdom and Ireland in 2008 by
Duncan Baird Publishers Ltd
Sixth Floor
Castle House
75–76 Wells Street
London W1T 3QH

Conceived, created and designed by
Duncan Baird Publishers

Managing Editor: Grace Cheetham
Editor: Dawn Bates
Managing Designer: Dan Sturges
Designer: Gail Jones
Commissioned photography: Toby Scott at Simon Smith studios

British Library Cataloguing-in-Publication Data:
A CIP record for this book is available from the British Library

ISBN: 978-1-84483-505-8

10 9 8 7 6 5 4 3 2 1

Typeset in Helvetica Condensed
Colour reproduction by Colourscan, Singapore
Printed in Thailand by Imago

Publisher's Note: The information in this book is not intended as a substitute for professional medical advice and treatment. If you are pregnant or breastfeeding or have any special dietary requirements, allergies or medical conditions, it is recommended that you consult a medical professional before following any of the information or recipes contained in this book. Duncan Baird Publishers, or any other persons who have been involved in working on this publication, cannot accept responsibility for any errors or omissions, inadvertent or not, that may be found in the recipes or text, nor for any problems that may arise as a result of preparing one of these recipes or following that advice contained in this work.

Notes on the recipes
Unless otherwise stated:
• Use medium eggs • Use fresh herbs • Do not mix metric and imperial measurements
• 1 tsp = 5ml, 1 tbsp = 15ml, 1 cup = 250ml • All recipes serve four.

CONTENTS

KEY TO SYMBOLS

- antioxidant
- antibacterial
- antiviral
- anti-inflammatory
- regulates hormones
- protects the heart
- anti-cancer
- anti-ageing
- good for the skin

Introduction

It really is possible to eat your way to good health and improve the way you feel and look. In *The Top 100 Health Tips* I've selected 100 delicious and nutritious foods that you can easily introduce into your diet for maximum impact on your health.

In Chapter 1, Health Improvers, discover what to eat to boost your immune system, soothe inflammation and speed up the healing process. The foods in Chapter 2, Detoxifiers and Digestion Soothers, help your digestion work more effectively, support the body's cleansing systems, combat ulcers and cure nausea. They can also solve disorders such as indigestion, constipation and irritable bowel syndrome. Chapter 3, Fitness Enhancers, includes eating strategies to provide sustained energy, improve performance, build and maintain strength, increase endurance and turn your food to muscle rather than fat. It also helps to reduce the risk of sports injuries and mineral imbalances. Chapter 4, Weight Shifters, is packed with tasty foods that fill you up sooner and for longer, combat hormonal weight gain and control blood-sugar. Some also help to burn off fat. Chapter 5, Brain Boosters and Mood Lifters, reveals how what you eat can improve your memory, libido, mood, sleeping patterns and mental alertness. It includes food to combat symptoms of PMS and the menopause. Chapter 6, Life Lengtheners, includes foods that combat chronic illness or conditions that strike in later life, such as cancers, heart disease, diabetes, arthritis, osteoporosis and prostate disease. They also help keep your eyes and skin young.

A VARIED DIET

Particular foods can be very effective against certain health conditions, but they shouldn't be eaten to the exclusion of other fresh produce. Most fruit and vegetables, especially, will do you good, and their benefits are too wide-ranging to be strictly categorized. The risk of heart disease and cancer is reduced by a particularly wide range of foods: see the symbols on each page.

Many health conditions stem from nutrient deficiencies, so they can be alleviated – and often cured – by eating better. Base your diet on a wide range of vegetables and fruits, backed by wholegrain cereals, organic meat and dairy products, with as little processed food as possible.

STORING FOOD

Fresh fruit and vegetables lose much of their vitamin content in storage. So shop where you know food is fresh, keep it in a fridge or a cool place and eat as soon as possible. Fresh herbs can be kept in a clean screwtop jar with a pinch of salt, covered with olive oil, or for a few days in the fridge, wrapped in damp paper. Fresh meat should be placed on a plate on the bottom shelf of the fridge, where it can't drip onto anything.

SUPPLEMENTS

It's always better to get your nutrients from a balanced diet, than by taking supplements. No one knows exactly how it works – only that the whole fruit or vegetable seems to provide a full range of nutrients in the right balance. Beta carotene, for example, is so good for the lungs that smokers who get plenty of it in their diet reduce their risk of lung cancer. Yet taking beta carotene supplements seems

STAR FOODS
Kale for your immune system (see page 16)
Mussels to combat inflammation (see page 26)
Apples for digestive health (see page 32)
Green beans for fitness (see page 52)
Garlic for weight loss (see page 70)
Tofu for fat burning (see page 76)
Sea vegetables to improve emotional health (see page 86)
Linseed to solve hormonal upheavals (see page 96)
Cherries for anti-ageing (see page 102)
Walnuts for your heart (see page 116)

to increase their cancer risk. It's almost impossible to overdose on the nutrients from fruit and vegetables, but it's easy to unbalance your levels of vitamins, and especially of minerals, if you take some of them in the large quantities supplied by supplements. The only exception is vitamin B12. Vegans who can't get enough of this from their diet should take this as part of a vitamin B-complex supplement.

EAT ORGANIC
Organic foods are produced in much the same way food was grown for thousands of years, until the twentieth century. Organic farmers don't use synthetic chemicals or sewage sludge. Their animals are given medicines only when they're unwell – not to make them put on weight faster or as a way of counteracting the unhealthy conditions of factory farms. Organic food has not been irradiated or genetically modified.

It's worth paying a little extra to eat organic, although the price difference is narrowing all the time. You'll avoid eating drug or chemical residues and have a much lower risk of catching a disease such as food poisoning from chicken. Not all scientific studies have found that organic foods are more nutritious, but many have – and none has found them less healthy! Animal welfare standards are higher, too, and organic farming is very much kinder to the environment. If you can't afford to buy all organic goods, prioritize meat products and out of season fruits and vegetables.

INGREDIENTS

Buy as much produce as possible that is in season. Fruit and vegetables are at their most nutritious during the season when they naturally grow, and when they are bought from local sources so that they are fresh when they reach you.

Stir-frying in a few millilitres of oil adds very little to the fat content, and helps the body to absorb fat-soluble vitamins such as A and D. Leafy vegetables can be steamed in a couple of minutes, often less.

FLEXIBLE RECIPES

Many recipes in this book are based on traditional dishes from around the world.

Feel free to adjust the quantities and substitute the ingredients to suit your individual taste. That's part of the pleasure of cooking. Salt is rarely mentioned: season to taste, but if you do usually add salt, just give the recipes a try without.

SAFETY WARNING

- Wash all fruit and vegetables. Non-organic should be well scrubbed or peeled; organic should be rinsed.
- Beansprouts must be extra carefully washed, as their growing conditions may encourage growth of microbes.
- Beans, especially kidney beans, can be poisonous if not properly cooked. Tinned beans are safe, easy and just as nutritious as the fresh version. If using dry beans, soak them for at least 5 hours, throw away the water and boil for 10 minutes. Then cook them for at least an hour in two to three times their volume of water. (Lentils don't need to be soaked beforehand.) Slow cookers don't get hot enough, and undercooked beans are even more poisonous than raw.
- Always clean seafood thoroughly, discarding any with shells that are broken or already open. When they are cooked, don't eat any that are still closed.
- Meat should be cooked through. Don't use too fierce a heat, though, as this can create chemical reactions that have been linked with cancer.
- Don't dry-fry anything in a non-stick pan.
- If you may have any health condition, do check with your doctor before changing your diet.

NUTRIENTS
Vitamins C, K; manganese; fibre

cranberry

Bacteria come unstuck when faced with these tiny, but tasty, infection-fighting fruits.

One of the natural-health success stories of the past few years, cranberries have proved their value in preventing urinary tract infections, such as cystitis. Many people now eat them every day, as a first line of defence against these painful and dangerous conditions. The powerful ingredient is a flavonoid called proanthocyanidins, which is more abundant in cranberries than in most other fruits. Proanthocyanidins prevent bacteria sticking to the urinary tract wall, and prevent infections of the mouth and stomach in the same way.

Soak dried fruit, such as currants and raisins, in cranberry juice for a tasty compote.

CRANBERRY SAUCE

115g/4oz/½ cup dried cranberries
250ml/9fl oz/1 cup cranberry
  or orange juice
2.5cm/1in root ginger, finely
  chopped
1 tbsp red wine (optional)
2 tbsp honey

Place the cranberries and juice in a pan and soak for 30 minutes. Bring to the boil, add the ginger and wine, if using, and simmer for 10 minutes, stirring. Mix in the honey and serve with meat or a nut roast.

kiwi fruit

The vitamin-filled strength of these refreshing fruits will keep you breathing freely.

Bite for bite, there is more vitamin C in a ripe kiwi fruit than in most citrus fruits. And although vitamin C is well known for warding off colds, its effects go much further than that. It protects the body from all kinds of infections and inflammation, and is particularly effective against respiratory diseases. Scientists have found that it helps reduce coughing, wheezing and rhinitis. People who eat kiwi fruit are less likely than others to suffer from asthma attacks, but it shouldn't be given to very small children as it can cause allergies. It is also good for the heart and vision. Eating kiwi fruits regularly has also been found to lower blood cholesterol and reduce the risk of blood clots.

NUTRIENTS

Vitamins C, E, beta carotene; copper, magnesium, potassium; fibre

KIWI AND AVOCADO SALAD

2 avocados, stoned and sliced
1 apple, cored and sliced
3 kiwi fruits, sliced
2 tsp lemon juice
3 tbsp olive oil
1 tbsp wine vinegar
100g/3½oz lettuce, shredded

Place the avocados, apple, 2 of the kiwi fruits and the lemon juice in a bowl and mix together. Crush the remaining kiwi fruit, blend with the olive oil and vinegar and pour over the fruit. Serve on a bed of lettuce.

orange

This popular fruit is best known for its vitamin C content, but it also contains many other disease-fighting compounds.

NUTRIENTS
Vitamins A, B1, C, folate; calcium, potassium; fibre

Oranges are known for their immune-boosting power. A medium-sized orange provides more than the average daily requirement of vitamin C, which fights off infections and strengthens the body's defences. Particularly effective against colds and other respiratory ailments, including asthma, oranges have also been found to reduce the risk of stomach ulcers, kidney stones and certain cancers. Their natural sugars help diabetics maintain their blood glucose levels. And a teaspoonful of grated organic orange peel added to food can reduce cholesterol. Citrus fruits also contain limonin, which is being researched for its anti-cancer and cholesterol-lowering possibilities.

ORANGE YOGURT SUNDAE

4 tbsp yogurt
zest of ½ orange, grated
2 oranges, sliced into wheels
1 banana, sliced
1 tbsp berries
¼ tsp cinnamon

Mix together the yogurt and the peel and chill for an hour. In a separate bowl, mix together the fruit and cinnamon and chill. Divide the fruit salad into bowls and spoon the yogurt over. Serve immediately.

raspberry

This tasty summer fruit may be small and delicate, but it has the power to protect against yeast infections and irritable bowel syndrome.

The flavonoids called anthocyanins that give a raspberry its exquisite colour are also responsible for some of its most valuable qualities. They have antimicrobial effects that can prevent the proliferation of bacteria and fungi in the digestive system. One of these, *Candida albicans*, causes the irritating vaginal infection called thrush and has also been linked with digestive disorders such as irritable bowel syndrome. Like all berries, raspberries are also packed with antioxidants that promote overall health in the long term. They protect eyesight, reduce the risk of certain cancers, and their soluble fibre content helps to keep blood-sugar levels steady.

NUTRIENTS
Vitamins B2, B3, C, folate; copper, magnesium, manganese, potassium; fibre

RASPBERRY SORBET

450g/1lb raspberries
juice and zest of 2 limes
2 tbsp honey

Place the raspberries in a blender and purée. Strain through a cloth into a bowl and discard the pulp.

Add the remaining ingredients and 250ml/9fl oz/1 cup water to the raspberries. Mix together well and freeze for 2–3 hours. Beat with a rolling pin or blend until it is a soft consistency, but not runny. Freeze again until set.

Brussels sprout

A small but powerful defender of the immune system, this crunchy vegetable easily punches above its weight in nutrients.

Brussels sprouts have huge health benefits. They are especially effective in supporting the immune system during the winter months when infections are most likely to strike. On top of their vitamin and mineral content, they contain numerous disease-fighting phytochemicals, including glucosinolates and antioxidant phenols. Glucosinolates are now believed to combat the carcinogens caused by overheating meat. Brussels sprouts are good for the skin too, giving it a healthy, lustrous glow.

NUTRIENTS

Vitamins B1, B2, B6, C, E, K, beta carotene, folate; calcium, copper, iron, magnesium, manganese, phosphorus, potassium; fibre; omega-3 oils; protein

---

BRUSSELS SPROUTS WITH CHESTNUTS

4 rashers bacon (optional)
400g/14oz Brussels sprouts, trimmed
400g/14oz chestnuts, cooked or vacuum-packed
25g/1oz butter
salt and pepper to taste

Grill the bacon, if using, and cut into strips. Steam or boil the sprouts for 5 minutes until cooked but still crunchy. Drain the sprouts, add the chestnuts, butter and the bacon strips, if using. Season and serve immediately.

carrot

This colourful vegetable may not actually make you see in the pitch dark, but it really is good for your eyes and overall vision.

The carrot is one of the richest sources of phytonutrients called carotenoids, which are responsible for its colour and for a host of health benefits. These nutrients are what make carrots so good for the eyes, particularly for seeing in poor light. Carrots have tough cell walls that do not give up their nutrients easily. To get the best nutritional value, they should be juiced or cooked rather than eaten raw. Cooking them with oil allows the body to use more beta carotene.

Eating just one carrot a day could halve a smoker's risk of lung cancer.

NUTRIENTS
Vitamins C, K, beta carotene; potassium; fibre

CARROTS IN ORANGE

450g/1lb carrots, cut
 into batons
1 tbsp olive oil
200g/7oz onions, chopped
1 tsp caraway seeds
4 tbsp orange juice

Parboil the carrots for 5 minutes, and drain. Heat the oil in a pan and sauté the onion for 3 minutes, then add the caraway seeds for 2 minutes. Add the carrots, pour the juice over and turn up the heat until the juice boils. Reduce the heat and simmer for 5 minutes, until most of the fluid has evaporated. Serve immediately.

kale

NUTRIENTS
Vitamins B6, C, E, K, beta carotene; calcium, copper, manganese, potassium; fibre

COLOURFUL KALE

450g/1lb carrots, cut into batons
225g/8oz frozen sweetcorn
450g/1lb kale leaves, roughly chopped
1 sweet pepper, deseeded and cut into strips
salt and pepper to taste

Place 500ml/18fl oz/2 cups water in a saucepan. Add the carrots, bring to the boil, then simmer for about 5 minutes. Add the frozen sweetcorn, kale and pepper, and simmer for a further 3 minutes. Season and serve immediately.

This leafy winter wonderfood will help to keep you healthy through the coldest time of the year.

Dark green leafy vegetables are highly nutritious, and kale is one of the top scorers. In winter your immune system comes under attack and this vitamin-C packed vegetable, providing your daily requirement in one large portion, is a potent defender against colds and viruses. Its anti-inflammatory effects also reduce the risk of asthma attacks and joint pains.

Kale in season has fewer pesticide residues, even if it is non-organic.

Weather-proof health

As well as boosting immunity, kale provides bone-building calcium to counteract the weakening effects of being less active in winter, and lutein and zeaxanthin, which will protect your eyes in wintry conditions. It contains plenty of fibre to keep blood-sugar levels steady, in case staying indoors during the cold weather tempts you to eat more. And all this comes for less than 45 calories a portion. Meanwhile, its long-term benefits as an antioxidant, cleansing and reducing the risk of cancer, are stacked up in your favour too.

Life-saver

Kale is exceptionally rich in beta carotene. If you're a smoker, or a passive smoker, it might just save your life. A compound in cigarette smoke has been found to cause vitamin A deficiency, which can lead to lung diseases including emphysema and cancer. But foods rich in beta carotene – which the body turns into vitamin A – can counteract these effects.

SESAME KALE

1 tbsp sesame oil
2 cloves garlic, crushed
450g/1lb kale leaves, roughly
   chopped
1 tsp soy sauce
1 tbsp toasted sesame seeds

Heat the oil in a pan and sauté the garlic for 30 seconds over a moderate heat. Add the kale leaves and 2 tablespoons of water and increase the heat, stirring frequently until the water has evaporated. Stir in the soy sauce and the sesame seeds just before serving.

onion

As strong in healing power as they are in taste, these vegetables keep disease at a safe distance.

The powerful anti-inflammatory effects of onions make them a vital ingredient in nourishing winter dishes. They are full of nutrients that counteract respiratory problems at all levels, from the nasal congestion caused by a cold to the wheezing of asthma. Their antibacterial action combats all kinds of infectious disease and they protect the digestive system, reducing the risk of intestinal growths that could lead to cancer. The same compounds cause the smell and the healing effects, so the more pungent the onion, the more good it will do you.

NUTRIENTS

Vitamins B6, C, folate; chromium, copper, manganese, molybdenum, phosphorus, potassium; fibre

ONION SOUP WITH CHEESY TOAST

4 tbsp olive oil
6 large onions, thinly sliced
2 tbsp flour
2 litres/70fl oz/8 cups stock
2 tbsp white wine
4 tbsp grated cheese
4 slices French bread

Heat the oil in a pan and fry the onions until golden. Stir in the flour. Add the stock gradually and bring to the boil, stirring all the while. Add the wine and simmer for 20 minutes. Sprinkle the cheese on the bread and toast under a grill. Pour the soup into bowls and place the toast on top. Serve immediately.

600

sweet pepper

This versatile vegetable provides an amazing array of nutrients to help you see clearly and breathe freely.

NUTRIENTS
Vitamins B6, C, K, beta carotene and other carotenoids

Peppers provide a healthy serving of immunity-boosting nutrients, including two antioxidants that work well together: beta carotene (the precursor of vitamin A) and vitamin C. Together, these offer protection against cell-damaging free radicals and protect the lungs from winter infections, asthma and even the ravages of second-hand smoke. Red peppers are especially high in cancer-fighting lycopene and in vitamin C and carotenoids, which protect vision and reduce the risk of eye diseases.

GRILLED PEPPER AND WALNUT SALAD

4 sweet peppers, deseeded
   and cut into strips
handful walnut halves
2 tbsp olive oil
1 tsp vinegar
1 lettuce, roughly torn
   salt to taste

Heat the peppers under a hot grill until the skin is black and blistered. When cool enough to touch, peel off the skin and discard. Heat the walnuts gently in 1 teaspoon of oil in a frying pan until crisp. Mix together the remaining oil, vinegar and salt. Place the lettuce in a serving bowl and the peppers and walnuts on top. Pour over the dressing and serve while still warm.

basil

This fragrant herb has antimicrobial effects that could reduce the risk of food poisoning.

Basil has long been used for healing: the Ayurvedic remedy tulsi is Holy basil (*Ocimum sanctum*), a close relative of our everyday Sweet basil (*Ocimum basilicum*). Basil leaves are rich in oils that reduce inflammation and kill harmful bacteria. Recent tests have found that these oils can counteract the growth of antibiotic-resistant superbugs, including those that cause food poisoning and others that infect wounds. As it was traditionally used as an anti-inflammatory remedy, its effects in that area are currently being studied. Around the house, a pot of basil is a traditional insect repellent.

NUTRIENTS

Vitamins A, C; calcium, iron, magnesium, manganese, potassium; fibre

Add the fresh leaves at the end of cooking to keep their flavour and their healthy effects.

TRICOLORE SALAD

450g/1lb cherry or napolina
tomatoes, halved
225g/8oz mozzarella, cubed
2 tbsp balsamic vinegar
generous handful basil leaves

Mix together the tomatoes and mozzarella in a serving bowl, pour over the vinegar and toss. Sprinkle the basil leaves on top and serve immediately.

clove

This fresh-tasting spice relieves toothache and sore mouths, and is a traditional remedy for bad breath.

Naturally antibacterial and anti-inflammatory, cloves are as likely to be found in herbal medicine chests as in the kitchen. They have long been used to numb the pain of toothache and, as well as having anaesthetic effects, they combat the bacterial infection and inflammation that can lead to gum disease and the risk of further damage to teeth. The oil in cloves contains a compound called eugenol that has long been used by dentists, and oil of cloves is still kept for that purpose in many homes. The anti-inflammatory properties of eugenol may protect other parts of the body, too, including joints.

NUTRIENTS
Vitamin C; calcium, magnesium, manganese; fibre; omega-3 oils

BAKED APPLES

- 4 heaped tbsp raisins or sultanas
- 1 tsp ground nutmeg
- 4 large unpeeled cooking apples, cored, skin scored around middle
- 4 tsp cloves
- 1 tbsp butter (optional)

Preheat the oven to 190°C/ 375°F/Gas 5. Mix the fruit with the nutmeg and stuff the mixture into each apple. Stud the skins with cloves and place on a greased baking tray. Pour 1 tablespoon of water over each apple and place a little butter on top, if using. Cook for 25 minutes or until soft, basting occasionally. Serve the apples on their own or with cream.

coriander

This versatile ingredient reduces the dangerous effects of hot weather on food.

NUTRIENTS
Iron, magnesium, manganese; fibre

EGYPTIAN GREENS SOUP

1 litre/35fl oz/4 cups stock
450g/1lb spinach, roughly
  torn
1 tbsp olive oil
4 tsp coriander seeds, ground
4 cloves garlic, crushed
½ tsp salt
1 tsp vinegar (optional)
2 tbsp finely chopped
  coriander leaves

Bring the stock to the boil in
a large pan. Add the spinach,
bring back to the boil and
simmer for 5 minutes. Heat
the oil in a frying pan and fry
the coriander seeds, garlic and
salt for 1–2 minutes, until the
garlic starts to brown. Add to
the spinach with the vinegar,
if using. Stir and sprinkle with
coriander. Serve immediately.

Coriander is unusual in that its leaves are used as a herb and its ground-up seeds as a spice. Both have long been popular among cooks in hot countries, especially where it is difficult to protect meat from heat and flies. Scientists have now discovered the reason behind the traditional lore: coriander offers protection against food poisoning. It contains antibacterial compounds that protect against numerous bugs, including some of the most dangerous, such as salmonella. Ayurvedic healers use coriander for its anti-inflammatory effects.

mustard

Valued for its warming effects, this plant has many ways of protecting the lungs.

Mustard seeds have long been used to relieve respiratory ailments. They are rich in selenium and magnesium, two key nutrients that are often lacking in modern diets, which both help to reduce inflammation in the lungs and ease the symptoms of asthma. A mustard-seed poultice on the chest may also help to rid the lungs of mucus. Less commonly used than the seeds, mustard leaves are rich in other nutrients, including vitamin C and beta carotene, that improve lung function and help protect against the harmful effects of second-hand tobacco smoke.

NUTRIENTS

Vitamin B3; calcium, iron, magnesium, manganese, phosphorous, selenium, zinc; fibre; omega-3 oils; protein

VINAIGRETTE DRESSING

2 tsp mustard seeds
1 tsp salt
2 cloves garlic (optional)
2 tbsp balsamic or wine vinegar
6 tbsp olive oil

Crush the mustard seeds with a pestle and mortar, or in a spice grinder, then add the salt and garlic, if using, and crush again. Transfer to a bowl, pour in the vinegar and olive oil and beat together.

NUTRIENTS

Vitamin B6; iron, manganese, potassium

Served with cruciferous vegetables, turmeric increases protection against prostate cancer.

turmeric

Prized for its colour, this spice is actually one of the most health-protective ingredients in a curry.

Many spices would have excellent effects if they were not eaten in such small quantities. Turmeric, however, is such a strong anti-inflammatory that the small amount used in a curry is enough to reduce the risk of illness. The potent ingredient is curcumin, which gives turmeric its vivid golden colour. It has been shown to protect against inflammatory bowel disease and several forms of cancer, relieve the pain and stiffness of arthritis and improve liver function. Turmeric may also counteract the carcinogenic effects of some additives that are found in processed food.

SPICED CAULIFLOWER

1 large cauliflower, broken into florets
1 tbsp groundnut oil
1 tsp ground coriander
1 tsp ground black pepper
1 large onion, chopped
1 tsp salt
1 tbsp turmeric

Steam the cauliflower for 10 minutes. Meanwhile, heat the oil in a pan over a low heat and briefly fry the coriander and black pepper. Add the onion and stir-fry for 3–5 minutes until translucent. Add the salt and turmeric. Stir in the cauliflower until well coated and serve.

chickpea

Rich in minerals that support the metabolic process, chickpeas keep you up to speed with a busy life.

The need for essential minerals, especially iron, increases when you're overworking, not least to help your body ward off infection. Women, in particular, tend to be deficient in iron until the menopause ends their monthly blood loss. If, like many people, you've cut down on red meat, you could be short of this vital mineral. Chickpeas, or garbanzos, provide plenty of iron, as well as helping to stabilize blood sugar. They also help the body deal with preservatives, found in some fast foods, that can cause headaches. Tinned chickpeas (without added sugar or salt) are just as nutritious as dried.

NUTRIENTS
Folate; copper, iron, manganese, molybdenum, phosphorus; fibre; protein

HUMMUS

400g/14oz tin chickpeas, drained
2 cloves garlic, crushed
3 tbsp lemon juice
2 tbsp tahini (sesame seed paste)
2 tbsp olive oil

Blend the chickpeas with the garlic and lemon juice, or mash them in a bowl. Stir in the tahini and oil and add a little water for smoothness, if wished. Serve with wholemeal bread or crudités.

mussel

NUTRIENTS
Vitamins B2, B6, B12, E, folate; iron, potassium, selenium, zinc

The dynamic duo of selenium and omega-3 fatty acids makes the often-overlooked mussel a nutritional superstar.

A weekly meal of mussels could help bring everyday ailments such as asthma, eczema and joint pain under control, and help to prevent hormonal upheaval. Mussels are rich in minerals, including selenium (hard to find in most diets), that reduce inflammation. Another powerful anti-inflammatory effect comes from omega-3 fatty acids, and mussels are richer in omega-3 than other shellfish. Both selenium and omega-3 help to regulate hormone production too. Omega-3's numerous good results include protecting

MUSSEL SOUP

1kg/2lb 4oz mussels, cleaned
1.5 litres/52fl oz/6 cups fish stock or water
1 tbsp olive oil
1 large onion, chopped
1 large carrot, diced
1 stick celery, chopped
125ml/4½fl oz/½ cup white wine
salt and pepper to taste

Boil the mussels in the stock in a covered pan until the shells open. Remove and discard the shells and any that haven't opened. Heat the oil and sauté the vegetables for 5 minutes. Strain the stock, then add to the vegetables. Add the wine, bring to the boil and simmer for 10 minutes until the vegetables are soft. Add the mussels, season and serve immediately.

MUSSELS WITH SALSA

4 tomatoes, diced
4 cloves garlic, crushed
2 small chillies, deseeded and chopped
2 green peppers, deseeded and chopped
juice of 2 lemons
2 tbsp olive oil

16 mussels, cleaned

To make the salsa, mix together all the ingredients, except for the mussels, and chill. Steam the mussels until the shells are all open. Serve with the salsa and fresh bread.

against cancer and heart disease, preventing cell damage and improving brain function.

The right choice

We're advised to eat oily fish 2–3 times a week, but some species are overfished, while others swim in polluted waters. Mussels, being sustainably farmed, offer a safe alternative. Follow the safety advice on page 9 when eating seafood.

Mussels contain twice as much iron, weight for weight, as red meat.

NUTRIENTS
Vitamins B2, B3, B6, B12; copper, iron, phosphorus, selenium, zinc; protein

VENISON MARINADE

2 tbsp olive oil
4 tbsp red wine
1 tbsp chopped rosemary
1 tbsp chopped thyme
4 cloves garlic, crushed
4 venison steaks

Mix together the oil, red wine, herbs and garlic in a bowl. Pour over the steaks in a non-metallic dish and marinate for at least an hour, turning occasionally. Grill the steaks under a moderate heat until cooked through. Serve immediately.

venison

For the strengthening and energy-boosting benefits of red meat with little fat, eat venison.

Meat from deer and their relatives is packed with protein, minerals and B vitamins. Because of the low fat content, it is much healthier than other red meat and is the ideal ingredient to boost depleted iron stores. Venison's abundant B vitamins help the body store energy and may protect against migraines. These vitamins play numerous other roles, too, such as protecting against bone disorders and certain cancers.

Venison is one of the richest sources of vitamin B12, which is hard to find except in meat.

⊙ ⚗ ◉ ✴ ♡ Ⓒ ⬤

honey

This versatile food will help to heal a wound, promote digestion and prevent mouth ulcers.

Honey has been used as a healing agent throughout history. Daubing an ulcer or wound with honey speeds recovery because of its antiseptic qualities and because it has a drying effect that inhibits the growth of fungi and bacteria. It can also reduce the risk of gum disease. Eating it is also valuable as it may improve digestion and recent research suggests that it can counteract food-poisoning bacteria. The bees' food sources affect the honey – its healing powers are increased if they feed on particularly healthy plants, such as the New Zealand manuka bush.

NUTRIENTS
Vitamins B2, B6; iron, manganese

HONEY VINAIGRETTE

2 tbsp honey
2 tbsp cider vinegar
3 tbsp extra virgin olive oil
1 tsp French mustard
    (optional)
pinch of salt

Pour the honey and vinegar into a pan and place over a low heat until just warm. Add the olive oil, beating the mixture with a fork. Remove from the heat, then add the mustard and salt. Serve with a warm salad, such as chicken.

⊙ ◑ ✋ ♡ C 👁 ⬤

lemon

NUTRIENTS
Vitamin C; flavonoids; limonin

Nothing tastes fresher than lemon, which has amazing cleansing and antioxidant powers.

Despite its sourness, lemon juice is a popular drink when diluted in water, with a cleansing taste few other fruits can match. During a brief detox fast, it quells the appetite and freshens breath. Used in a marinade or dressing, lemon aids digestion by breaking down some of the tough components of meat. Its calming effects on the digestive system relieve bloating and heartburn. It also has a slightly antibacterial effect, reducing the risk of discomfort in the intestines. Packed with vitamin C, lemon's powerful antioxidant effects strengthen all the body's cells, aiding detoxification.

TANGY FISH

4 skinless tuna or other fish fillets
zest and juice of 1 lemon
zest and juice of 1 lime
2 tbsp olive oil
2 tsp finely chopped chives
1 tsp ground black pepper

Preheat the grill and place the fish on a foil-lined grill pan. Mix the zests with the oil and coat each fish fillet. Grill for around 8–10 minutes, until cooked through, turning once. Mix together the juices, chives and pepper. Pour the mixture over the fish and serve immediately.

prune

Dried plums regulate the digestive system, speeding it up or slowing it down – whichever is needed.

Containing many of the same nutrients as fresh plums, prunes also have a beneficial effect on the digestive system. They have long been used as the most effective, yet gentle, natural remedy for constipation. Their fibre-rich bulk softens food waste that has dried out during an excessive delay in the colon, and helps it move painlessly on and out of the body. Yet they may also slow the movement of food from the stomach if it is emptying too quickly, causing indigestion or wind. Prunes lower cholesterol by helping the body to excrete fats, and feed the good bacteria in the intestine, helping to prevent harmful bacteria breeding.

NUTRIENTS
Beta carotene; copper, potassium; fibre

DRIED FRUIT COMPOTE

2 heaped tbsp chopped prunes
2 tbsp chopped dried apple
2 tbsp dried berries or other dried fruit
1 tsp lemon juice

Put all the ingredients in a bowl and cover with water. Refrigerate overnight. Stir well and serve for breakfast, topped with yogurt.

021

apple

NUTRIENTS
Vitamins C, K; fibre; flavonoids

This fruit works wonders for both detox and digestion thanks to the combination of pectin and fibre.

Apples have a huge number of health benefits, and scientists are only just starting to identify their numerous life-enhancing nutrients, but their superstar role is in digestion and detoxification. Eating an apple aids a detox by helping you feel full sooner and for longer, and can alleviate even chronic constipation, a widespread problem often caused by poor nutrition. Constipation prevents the body getting rid of toxins and can lead to more serious conditions, from haemorrhoids to colon cancer.

Gentle gel

Apples are rich in soluble and insoluble fibre, both of which help food progress at a healthy pace through the digestive system. These fibres pick up toxic waste, such as heavy metals, along the way – as well as cholesterol, which is one reason why apples are also good for the arteries. The toxins and cholesterol can then be safely excreted, with the help of the soluble fibre, pectin. It forms a gel-like substance that softens the body's waste and helps it leave the body naturally. Pectin has a regulating effect on the speed of digestion, slowing it down as

---

APPLE CHARLOTTE

1kg/2lb 4oz cooking apples, cored and sliced
2 tbsp honey
½ tsp cinnamon
pinch of nutmeg
8 slices bread, buttered both sides

Pre-heat the oven to 190°C/375°F/Gas 5. Heat the apples with 2 tablespoons of water in a pan, stirring until a thick purée. Stir in the honey, cinnamon and nutmeg. Line the sides and base of a greased cake tin with half the bread, spoon the purée in and top with the other half. Bake for 30 minutes, until it is golden brown. Serve immediately.

well as speeding it up when necessary. Its gel-like effects can also alleviate diarrhoea, which removes food from the system too quickly for vital nutrients to be absorbed and can lead to dangerous levels of dehydration.

Apple peel is also rich in quercetin, which reduces the risk of sun damage to skin.

artichoke

This spiky little plant could hold a soothing answer to irritable bowel syndrome.

The rich fibre content of artichoke aids digestion. If you suffer from indigestion or irritable bowel syndrome, artichoke may relieve symptoms such as abdominal pain, flatulence, nausea, constipation and diarrhoea. It works by stimulating the flow of bile, a substance that helps to digest fat and encourages healthy movement of the intestine. This also prevents toxins building up in the liver and reduces the risk of gallstones. Eating an artichoke can reduce the effects of eating rich food.

NUTRIENTS
Vitamins B6, C; calcium, iron, magnesium, manganese, phosphorus, potassium; fibre

FRESH ARTICHOKE

4 globe artichokes, outer leaves and stalk removed
8 tbsp vinaigrette (see page 23)

Boil the artichokes in salted water for 30–40 minutes until you can pull off the leaves easily. Drain and leave to cool. To eat, pull off the leaves and dip into the vinaigrette. Bite off the fleshy part with your teeth and discard the leaf. Cut out the hairy 'choke' and eat the heart.

beetroot

The nutrient that gives beetroot its distinctive colour has detoxifying and cancer-fighting powers.

The brilliant ruby hue of beetroot has given it a traditional reputation as a blood cleanser. It certainly aids cell cleansing by increasing the liver's production of detoxifying enzymes, and the betacyanin that makes beetroot red is particularly effective in combating cancerous changes, too. Beetroot is a popular component of juice fasts, when mixed with a sweeter juice such as apple to dilute the taste. Scientists have found that the juice combats the effects of nitrates – chemical preservatives in processed meats that can cause colon cancer.

NUTRIENTS

Vitamin C, folate; copper, iron, magnesium, manganese, potassium, phosphorus; fibre

BEETROOT SOUP

2 tbsp olive oil
1 onion, chopped
2 cloves garlic, crushed
4 large beetroots, chopped
2 carrots, chopped
1 litre/35fl oz/4 cups stock
4 tbsp yogurt

Heat the oil in a large pan and gently fry the onion for 2–3 minutes, then add the garlic and cook for another minute. Add the beetroots, carrots and stock and bring to the boil. Cover and simmer gently for about 45 minutes, until cooked. Purée, then divide into bowls and top with yogurt.

broccoli

A potent defender against stomach ulcers, broccoli banishes harmful bacteria.

NUTRIENTS
Vitamins A, B6, C, E, K, folate; magnesium, phosphorus, potassium; fibre

As well as aiding the body's detoxification processes, broccoli is rich in a compound called sulphoraphane, which strengthens the ability of cells to resist damage. It has recently been found to improve digestion by fighting the unusually tough bacterium *Helicobacter pylori*. Not only does this bacterium thrive in the stomach acid that kills most bacteria, but it can even, in some cases, withstand antibiotics. Eating away at the stomach lining, it creates ulcers that can develop into cancer. Broccoli counteracts the painful effects, and may even reduce the amount of harmful bacteria in the stomach.

BROCCOLI WITH ALMONDS

450g/1lb broccoli florets
1 tsp olive oil
55g/2oz flaked almonds
juice of 1 lemon
2 tbsp broccoli sprouts (optional)

Steam the broccoli florets for 5–10 minutes until they are just tender. Meanwhile, heat the olive oil in a pan over a low heat and fry the flaked almonds until brown. Mix together the broccoli and almonds in a serving dish and sprinkle the lemon juice over. Top the dish with broccoli sprouts, if using.

025

cauliflower

These delicate florets provide powerful back-up for the liver in cleansing the body.

One of the cruciferous family of vegetables, cauliflower has many health-giving attributes, including the ability to aid cell detoxification. Processed food is full of manufactured chemicals, and even healthy food can contain elements that have harmful side effects if they linger in the body. The liver works hard to filter out these toxins, which can cause cell damage leading to cancer and other diseases, and is helped by cauliflower, which is rich in antioxidants. But cauliflower's most powerful effects come from compounds, such as glucosinolates, that fuel and strengthen the liver during all stages of detoxification.

NUTRIENTS
Vitamins B5, B6, C, folate; manganese; fibre; omega-3 oils

One large serving of cauliflower provides all the vitamin C you need in a day.

CAULIFLOWER PROVENÇALE

1 tbsp olive oil
1 large onion, chopped
2 cloves garlic, crushed
2 small courgettes, diced
400g/14oz tin tomatoes
1 large cauliflower, cut
   into florets

Heat the oil and fry the onion for 2–3 minutes. Stir in the garlic, add the courgettes and tomatoes and simmer for 5–10 minutes. Meanwhile, steam the cauliflower for 5–10 minutes until tender and place in a serving dish. Pour over the sauce and serve.

cucumber

This crunchy salad vegetable, packed with mineral-rich fluid, aids digestion by keeping you hydrated.

The rich fibre content of cucumbers keeps the digestive system moving and, unlike some other high-fibre foods, comes balanced with its own supply of fluid. Eating cucumbers can ease or prevent constipation, which is often caused by not drinking enough. It's helpful, too, if you've had diarrhoea, because as well as rehydrating it replaces vital minerals. Fresh cucumber juice can also alleviate acid indigestion. Cucumber's minerals are clustered in the peel, but the flesh, famed for soothing irritated skin, is rich in vitamin C and caffeic acid, which reduces inflammation.

NUTRIENTS

Vitamins A, C, folate; magnesium, manganese, molybdenum, potassium, silica; fibre

CUCUMBER AND MINT SALAD

4 tbsp chopped mint, plus
  a few leaves for garnish
1 large cucumber, chopped
2 sticks celery, chopped
2 tsp white wine vinegar
8 tbsp low-fat yogurt

Mix together the chopped mint, cucumber and celery in a serving bowl. In a separate bowl whisk the vinegar into the yogurt. Pour the dressing over the salad, garnish with mint leaves and serve.

curly endive

This traditional remedy may taste bitter, but it has sweetly soothing effects on digestion.

These distinctive leaves contain intybin, which stimulates the appetite and prepares the digestive system to cope with rich food. It is this compound that gives curly endive its slightly bitter taste (the sharper the taste, the greater the benefits), and makes it an appetizing first course. Curly endive also has detoxifying effects, acting as a tonic to the liver and gallbladder. Its diuretic actions help the body eliminate toxins through increased urination. Its relatives (including other endives, chicories and raddichio) have some of the same effects.

NUTRIENTS
Vitamins A, B-complex, beta carotene; iron, potassium

SUPER STARTER

4 curly endive leaves, shredded
4 red radicchio leaves, shredded
2 small chicory, separated
2 pears, cored and diced
8 shelled walnuts
honey vinaigrette (see page 29)

Toss all the ingredients together and dress with some honey vinaigrette. Serve immediately.

watercress

The peppery taste of these dark leaves gives a hint of their stimulating power.

NUTRIENTS
Vitamins B1, B6, C, E, K, beta carotene, folic acid; calcium, iron, zinc; protein

Packed with nutrients, watercress has long been valued for its medicinal properties. It is a mild diuretic, preventing the discomfort of fluid retention by helping the kidneys pass more urine. As a traditional cleansing remedy, it is considered to support liver function and purify the blood – with improved skin quality as a visible result. Scientists have just started understanding its truly detoxifying effects: watercress contains some of the strongest anti-cancer nutrients found in plants. These compounds – including phenylethylisothiocyanate, or PEITC, which gives watercress its distinctive peppery taste – help in two stages of cell detoxification by rendering carcinogens harmless.

STIR-FRIED WATERCRESS WITH ALMONDS AND GINGER

4 tbsp flaked almonds
2 tbsp sesame oil
450g/1lb watercress, chopped
5cm/2in root ginger, finely
   chopped
4 tbsp miso
4 tbsp rice vinegar

Heat a wok or pan and briefly dry- fry the almonds, then set aside. Add the oil to the wok and stir-fry the watercress and ginger for 3 minutes. Add the miso, rice vinegar and the almonds, stir well and serve immediately.

black pepper

This underrated spice has a dual action in speeding toxins out of the body through sweat and urine.

Black pepper aids digestion and detoxification in several ways. Its spicy taste stimulates the taste buds, encouraging the body to secrete more hydrochloric acid, which breaks food down in the stomach. If the body doesn't produce enough hydrochloric acid, food may stay in the stomach for too long, causing feelings of indigestion. Or it may be only partly digested when it moves on into the intestines, where it will produce wind and may lead to diarrhoea. Black pepper's action promotes complete digestion. Peppery foods also increase the production of urine, in which toxins filtered by the kidneys are removed from the body. And pepper's warming effects increase sweating, another route for elimination.

NUTRIENTS

Vitamin K; iron, manganese; fibre

Black pepper is believed to speed up fat burning by stimulating metabolic processes.

BLACK PEPPER RICE

350g/12oz/1¾ cups
   basmati rice, cooked
2 tbsp black peppercorns
2 tsp mustard seeds
2 tbsp groundnut oil
115g/4oz cashew nuts
½ tsp turmeric

Cook the rice for 10 minutes. Dry-fry the peppercorns and seeds for 2 minutes. Grind in a pestle and mortar. Heat the oil, add the nuts and turmeric and stir-fry for 2 minutes. Stir in peppercorns, seeds and rice. Serve.

NUTRIENTS
Iron, manganese

CUMIN CARROTS

1 tbsp cumin seeds
450g/1lb carrots, cut into
    batons
1 tbsp nut oil
2 cloves garlic, crushed
2 tbsp white wine

Dry-fry the seeds briefly in a
pan and grind in a pestle and
mortar or spice grinder. Boil
the carrots for 5 minutes until
nearly tender and drain. Heat
the oil in the pan and sauté
the garlic for 1 minute. Add
the wine and carrots and cook
until the wine has evaporated.
Stir in the cumin and serve
immediately.

cumin seed

This tasty spice has a distinctive warm fragrance
and is an effective digestive aid.

Cumin has long been valued in Asia and the Middle East for its
digestive benefits. It relieves wind and may prevent digestive
upsets such as diarrhoea. Medical science has now suggested
a reason why: these small seeds – greenish-brown, black and
white – may stimulate the production of pancreatic enzymes
that help the body break down foods and absorb the nutrients.
It kills many food-borne bacteria and supports the liver in its
detoxifying processes. Chewing a few seeds sweetens the breath
after eating meat. End a meal by chewing a blend of cumin seeds,
fennel, cloves and cardamom to enhance digestion.

ginger

The best and gentlest remedy for nausea, this is a mainstay for travellers and pregnant women.

Keeping ginger biscuits to hand during early pregnancy is a piece of advice that's been handed down for generations. Ginger has now been recognized by scientists as a fast-acting cure for nausea of all kinds, more effective than routinely used drugs. It's also a traditional cure for indigestion. Ginger's warming effects promote detoxification by increasing sweat. It is also a powerful anti-inflammatory that can relieve the pain of arthritis and its active ingredients, gingerols, can kill cancer cells. For strongest effects, pour hot water on a thumb-sized piece of peeled, crushed fresh root and drink it as a tea.

NUTRIENTS
Vitamin B6; copper, magnesium, manganese, potassium

SWEET AND SOUR VEGETABLES

1 large onion, chopped
2 tbsp nut oil
2 cloves garlic, crushed
5cm/2in root ginger, finely chopped
4 tbsp apple juice
900g/2lb non-root vegetables of choice, chopped
2 tbsp soy sauce

Heat the oil in a wok and fry the onion for 2–3 minutes. Add the garlic, ginger and apple juice. Cook for 3 minutes. Add the vegetables and stir-fry until tender. Stir in the soy sauce just before serving.

032

peppermint

This popular and fragrant herb has soothing effects on the muscles of the digestive system.

From a bunch of fresh leaves to a tube of sweets, any form of peppermint can relieve digestive upsets fast. It soothes the burning pain of indigestion, kills bacteria, relieves wind and regulates intestinal movement. Its ability to stop muscle spasm makes it a useful remedy for irritable bowel syndrome and for the abdominal cramps felt during painful periods. Use it with caution if you suffer from heartburn (when stomach acids rise into the throat) as although peppermint helps many sufferers, others find that it makes heartburn worse.

NUTRIENTS

Vitamins A, B2, C, folate; calcium, copper, iron, magnesium, manganese, potassium; fibre; omega-3 oils

Garnish salads and cooked foods with fresh mint leaves to aid digestion.

MINT TEA

4 tbsp finely chopped peppermint
2.5cm/1in root ginger, finely chopped
2 tsp honey

Boil 500ml/18fl oz/2 cups water and pour over the mint and ginger. Leave to steep until cool enough to drink. Stir in the honey and drink when dissolved.

yogurt

This stomach-soothing food can provide dairy benefits to people who can't drink milk.

Some people are unable to digest dairy products because their body doesn't produce an enzyme called lactase. However, because the culture in yogurt produces its own lactase it can be enjoyed by most people. Yogurt also promotes the growth of beneficial bacteria in the intestines. Probiotic yogurts aim to help even more by having the starter culture still alive, and are sometimes supplemented with other cultures. Eating yogurt can combat the bacterium that causes stomach ulcers.

NUTRIENTS
Vitamins B2, B5, B12; calcium, iodine, molybdenum, phosphorus, potassium, zinc; protein

Eating yogurt can reduce the risk of catching stomach bugs while on holiday.

YOGURT WITH NUTS AND HONEY

400g/14oz/1½ cups yogurt
handful walnut halves
4 tbsp runny honey
4 tbsp almonds

Mix the yogurt with the walnuts in a bowl. Drizzle the honey in a spiral around the top. Sprinkle with almonds and serve.

NUTRIENTS
Vitamins B1, B6, C; manganese, potassium; flavonoids

> A combination of grapes and bite-size cheese cubes make a great post-workout reviver.

grape

This juicy and refreshing fruit is easy to snack on – it is energizing and replaces the essential minerals you lose during a workout.

When fitting in food before exercise is a problem, grapes provide a refreshing solution. Exercising soon after a meal is a recipe for indigestion, but if you work out on an empty stomach you'll have little energy to use. Grapes, an ideal pre-workout snack, are light, rich in quick-energy carbohydrate and easily digestible, and they replenish some of the fluid and minerals you'll lose as you sweat. It helps if you can keep them in your pocket and nibble them as you go along. Grapes also keep your heart strong by lowering harmful cholesterol.

REFRESHING GRAPE SALAD

1 tsp olive oil
1 tbsp wine vinegar
2 apples, cored and chopped
110g/4oz seedless grapes
1 small cucumber, chopped

Mix together the oil and vinegar in a bowl to make a dressing. Mix together the apples, grapes and cucumber, pour the dressing over and serve.

pineapple

A versatile enzyme in this refreshing fruit can help to heal the aches, pains and bruises that often result from playing sports.

NUTRIENTS
Vitamins B1, B6, C; copper, manganese; fibre

Snacking on pineapple can help the body to heal faster, thanks to the plentiful nutrients it contains. One enzyme in particular, called bromelain, works as a powerful anti-inflammatory. It reduces the risk of inflammation when joints and muscles have been overworked or suffered minor damage. Backed by pineapple's rich vitamin C content, it also helps the body heal faster from bumps and bruises. The same action eases the pain of inflammatory conditions such as arthritis and sore throats. Fresh pineapple is most effective, as processing reduces bromelain's strength.

PINEAPPLE SALSA

1 small pineapple
1 red onion, diced
1 tsp lemon juice
5cm/2in root ginger, finely chopped
1 tbsp chopped mint

Remover the outer skin and chop the pineapple. Mix in the onion, lemon juice, ginger and mint. Chill for up to 12 hours. Serve with cold meats or fish.

watermelon

Much more than just the juiciest way to rehydrate after a workout, this refreshing fruit wards off any ill effects of exercise.

NUTRIENTS
Vitamins B1, B6, C, beta carotene; potassium, magnesium; lycopene

Watermelon contains minerals that help your body use its fluid most effectively, but it's doing far more than just replenishing fluid. It gives a healthy dose of energizing B vitamins to keep you going. Packed with anti-inflammatory vitamin C, it also helps to soothe overworked body tissues. And it is rich in lycopene, a powerful antioxidant that can prevent the cell damage caused by free radicals released during exercise. Unlike many fruits, watermelon loses little of its nutritional value when it's cut, so slices can be kept in the fridge for a few days.

WATERMELON REVIVER

4 unwaxed oranges
8 tbsp yogurt
4 bananas, sliced
250g/8oz watermelon, chopped

Grate the orange peel and mix the zest with the yogurt. Peel the oranges and slice into wheels. Layer the oranges and bananas in 4 glass bowls. Top with the watermelon and pour over the yogurt mixture. Serve.

alfalfa sprout

All types of sprouts are nutritious and energy-giving, but the tiny, delicate alfalfa variety is the best of a very good bunch.

Packed with nutrients, sprouts provide a burst of energy to see you through a workout. Alfalfa is one of the most nutritious, and it contains a compound that inhibits fungal growth, an occasional by-product of sweaty environments. Alfalfa sprouts are an unusually concentrated source of nutrients. The exact content of other sprouts varies according to the kind of bean they sprouted from, but all are nutritious. Rich in enzymes and fibre, they are easy to digest and contain very few calories.

NUTRIENTS

Vitamins B-complex, C, D, E, K; calcium, iron, potassium, zinc; fibre

SPROUT SALAD

8 large lettuce leaves
250g/8oz alfalfa sprouts
4 sticks celery, chopped
1 large cucumber, diced
4 tbsp vinaigrette (see page 23)
4 tbsp seeds or nuts

Line 4 bowls with the lettuce leaves. Wash the sprouts and add the celery and cucumber. Pour over the vinaigrette dressing, sprinkle over the seeds or nuts, and serve.

FITNESS ENHANCERS

celery

This crunchy fitness snack counteracts the dangers of drinking too much water during a workout.

A stick of celery is the athlete's secret weapon because it's rich in a string of nutrients that keep energy levels high. It's an excellent source of vitamin C, which aids recovery from sports injuries by strengthening cell walls. Celery also has a slightly diuretic effect. And being higher in sodium than most vegetables (though nowhere near a harmful level), celery could prevent the dangerous mineral imbalance that results from drinking too much water during an energetic workout.

Sticks of celery stuffed with fromage frais or low-fat soft cheese makes a great snack on the run.

NUTRIENTS
Vitamins B1, B2, B6, C, beta carotene, folic acid; calcium, iron, magnesium, manganese, molybdenum, phosphorus potassium; fibre

CELERY AND BLUE CHEESE SALAD

1 tbsp lemon juice
1 tbsp olive oil
½ tsp salt
2 apples, cored and chopped
2 sticks celery, chopped
1 bulb fennel, sliced
55g/2oz blue cheese, such as Stilton, diced

Mix together the juice, oil and salt. Pour over the apples, celery and fennel and top with cheese. Serve immediately with crusty bread.

○ ♡ ⓒ

potato

This staple vegetable is packed with vitamins and other energizing nutrients.

Don't overlook the value of potatoes if you're aiming to get fit. They're rich in vitamin B6, which – among many other essential services – is needed to mobilize the body's glycogen stores and help protein to build muscle. They are also packed with complex carbohydrates, the best form of energy food. Complex carbs play two roles, both essential to fitness. By providing slow-burning fuel, they give you enough energy to complete your workout without flagging halfway through. And they help the body to maintain the muscle it has built. Peeling removes many nutrients, so eat potatoes in their skins.

NUTRIENTS
Vitamins B6, C; copper, manganese potassium; fibre

TUNISIAN POTATOES WITH EGGS

4 eggs
450g/1lb potatoes, diced
juice of 1 lemon
2 tbsp cumin
2 tbsp olive oil
½ tsp harissa

Boil the eggs for 10 minutes. Leave to cool, then peel and chop. Boil the potatoes for 5–10 minutes until tender, and drain. Mix together the remaining ingredients and pour over the potatoes. Place on top of the eggs and serve immediately.

green bean

These nutritional power-packs hold many benefits for anyone taking exercise.

Runner beans and their close relatives, string or French beans, are a rich source of the nutrients required for exercise. Although each of these nutrients is valuable individually, their powers are multiplied when many are contained in one food. The kind of range found in green beans allows them to work together in building and maintaining peak fitness. The vitamin K content, for example, promotes the healing of scrapes and cuts, while vitamin C backs this up by maintaining the strength of cell walls. The B vitamins work together to keep nerves functioning well and energy levels high.

Eat the freshest young green beans – straight from the plant is best.

GREEN BEAN SALAD

2 eggs (optional)
200g/7oz waxy potatoes, diced
150g/5oz green beans, trimmed
juice of ½ lemon
1 tbsp walnut oil
black pepper to taste

Boil the eggs, if using, for 10 minutes. Boil the potatoes for 5–10 minutes and drain. Blanch the beans in boiling water and remove while still crisp. Peel and chop the eggs, if using, and mix together with the potatoes and beans, when cool. Mix the lemon juice and oil, and pour over the salad. Season with pepper and serve.

Pumping iron

Green beans are packed with essential minerals: manganese and magnesium contribute towards building and maintaining bone strength; iron is a vital nutrient that health-conscious people who avoid eating fatty animal foods may lack; and zinc helps to build strong bones, while speeding up recovery from muscular injuries. Cardiovascular fitness is central to any exercise regime: you're not only protecting your heart but also increasing its capacity to keep you going. Many of the nutrients in green beans work together to keep blood vessels strong, flexible and unimpeded by cholesterol deposits. This allows blood to move oxygen and nutrients around your body fast, keeping you at peak strength and energy.

CHINESE BEANS

450g/1lb green beans, cut
    into finger-length pieces
1 tbsp groundnut oil
1 garlic clove, crushed
5cm/2in root ginger, finely
    chopped
1 tbsp peanuts, chopped
1 tbsp soy sauce

Steam the beans until they are just tender and set aside. Heat the groundnut oil and briefly stir-fry the garlic and ginger. Add the beans and peanuts and stir-fry for 2–3 minutes to heat through. Add the soy sauce and serve immediately.

spinach

Eat this powerful vegetable for strength, energy and endurance. It guarantees you will be fighting fit.

The strength of spinach lies in its rich content of a large number of nutrients that work together. It is an excellent source of iron, but is equally rich in vitamin C, which helps the body to use iron efficiently. Similarly with calcium, magnesium and vitamin K, which all help build and maintain bone strength. It's a myth that the oxalate content prevents the body absorbing calcium: it just contains far more calcium than the oxalates can bind. Just 2 tablespoons of cooked spinach contain more than the daily requirement of vitamin K and most of the beta carotene you need.

NUTRIENTS

Vitamins B2, B3, B6, C, E, K, beta carotene, folic acid; calcium, copper, magnesium, manganese, iron, phosphorus, potassium, selenium, zinc; fibre; omega-3 oils; protein; tryptophan

EASY EGGS FLORENTINE

450g/1lb spinach
½ tsp vinegar
4 eggs
4 tbsp grated cheese
black pepper to taste

Put the spinach in a pan with the lid on tightly and cook over a low heat for 2 minutes until wilted. Bring a pan of water to the boil and add the vinegar. Carefully break the eggs into the water and poach them for 3 minutes. Put the spinach in a baking dish and place the eggs on top. Sprinkle cheese over and melt under a grill. Season and serve as it is or on toast.

black bean

It's no wonder people say you're 'full of beans' when they can see you've got energy to spare.

When you're working out regularly, it's important to eat high-protein foods that build and preserve muscle. As vegetarians know, this doesn't have to be meat. Beans are a healthy alternative, providing a dose of protein with a very low fat content. Black beans are also rich in nutrients, such as iron, that increase energy levels, which in turn helps to feed the muscles with oxygen. They are also packed with soluble fibre to stabilize blood sugar and maintain stamina. Beans with brown rice is an ideal meat-free protein-rich meal.

NUTRIENTS
Vitamin B1, folic acid; iron, magnesium, manganese, molybdenum, phosphorus; fibre; protein

EASY BLACK BEANS

2 sweet potatoes, chopped
2 tbsp groundnut oil
2 onions, roughly chopped
1 tsp cumin
4 cloves garlic, crushed
2 sweet peppers, deseeded
 and diced
400g/14oz tin black beans,
 drained

Boil the potatoes for 10–15 minutes. Reserve the water. Heat the oil and fry the onions for 2–3 minutes. Add the cumin and garlic, and cook for 1 minute. Add the peppers and cook for 3 minutes. Add the beans and 4 tablespoons of sweet-potato water. Bring to the boil and simmer for 5 minutes, adding the potato for the final minute. Serve.

lentil

Packed with minerals and complex carbohydrates, lentils build strength and endurance.

NUTRIENTS

Vitamin B1, folic acid; copper, iron, manganese, molybdenum, phosphorus, potassium; fibre; protein

DHAL

1 tbsp groundnut oil
1 tsp mustard seeds
1 large onion, finely chopped
2 cloves garlic, crushed
1 tsp ground cumin
2.5cm/1in root ginger, finely
    chopped
200g/7oz/¾ cup lentils

Heat the oil and fry the mustard seeds until they pop. Add the onion, garlic, cumin and ginger and stir-fry for 3–5 minutes until the onion is softened. Add the lentils and 625ml/27fl oz/3 cups water and bring to the boil. Simmer for 30-40 minutes. Serve with bread or rice, or refrigerate overnight.

It's vital to choose the right kind of snack before exercising. Lentils provide the perfect combination of nutrients to allay hunger pangs and spark long-lasting energy. A spoonful of dhal on bread, for example, is sustaining but not heavy, so it won't slow you down or cause indigestion. Lentils are rich in complex carbohydrates, which the body turns into glucose, providing a steady source of energy. They also contain iron, and plenty of protein with very little fat.

Lentils help improve blood circulation, keeping muscles oxygenated during exercise.

044

pumpkin seed

These nutritious nibbles help your joints, heart and circulation keep up when you're keeping fit.

Exercise requires good circulation, and pumpkin seeds are rich in a compound that could help. Pumping oxygenated blood rapidly around the body puts pressure on the arteries, which need to remain flexible and clear. Pumpkin seeds are one of the richest natural sources of phytosterols, which reduce the risk of arteries becoming narrowed by cholesterol. As well as being a rich source of many minerals, they contain omega-3 oils, which are anti-inflammatory and protect joints from damage during high-impact activities, and promote healing if you get injured while playing sports or exercising.

NUTRIENTS
Vitamin K; copper, iron, magnesium, manganese, phosphorus, zinc; omega-3 oils; protein

VEGAN PESTO

115g/4oz/ ¾ cup pumpkin
   seeds
4 cloves garlic
2 tbsp olive oil
generous handful basil leaves
1 tsp ground black pepper

Blend the seeds, garlic and oil in a food processor until well mixed. Add more oil for a smoother texture. Add the basil and blend. Add the pepper and serve with freshly cooked pasta.

045

NUTRIENTS
Vitamins B1, B6, E, folic acid; magnesium, manganese, zinc

A handful of wheat germ trail mix provides endurance and energy when you're hiking.

TRAIL MIX

1 tbsp pumpkin or sunflower seeds
1 tsp sesame seeds
2 tsp flaked almonds
1 tbsp wheat germ
1 tbsp raisins
1 tbsp finely chopped dried apricots

Mix together all the seeds and nuts and shake well. Mix in the wheat germ, raisins and dried apricots. Eat as a snack or serve on cereal.

wheat germ

This grain gives the energizing benefits of whole cereal, without causing an energy spike and slump.

Wheat germ is the heart of the cereal, containing many of its most valuable nutrients. It's rich in powerful antioxidants called phenolics, which protect the cells from damage that can be caused by exercise. It also contains cysteine, which helps keep the lungs clear and functioning at their peak. Its other vitamins and minerals contribute to boosting energy and endurance. Wholemeal bread and flour contain wheat germ. But it is missing from white bread and standard baking products, which is why these provide a quick energy rush followed by a slump.

cashew nut

This instant and nutritious snack replenishes mineral supplies while you burn off the fat.

NUTRIENTS

Copper, magnesium, phosphorus; monounsaturated fats; tryptophan

There is no handier snack than a packet of nuts when you've worked up an appetite exercising. Cashews are packed with minerals essential to fitness: magnesium keeps bones strong while combating muscle fatigue and soreness; copper not only increases energy and protects joints from injury, but also helps the body to utilize iron. You're still burning calories fast an hour or so after a workout, so enjoy some cashews rather than an empty-calorie snack. They're rich in monounsaturated fats, which bring a lot of heart-strengthening benefits.

CHICKEN WITH CASHEWS

1 tbsp groundnut oil
2 bird's eye chillies, deseeded and chopped
5cm/2in root ginger, finely chopped
450g/1lb marinated chicken (see page 60), cubed
2 spring onions, chopped
2 tsp vinegar
2 tsp sesame oil
2 heaped tbsp cashew nuts

Heat the groundnut oil and briefly stir-fry the chillies and ginger. Add the chicken and stir-fry for 2–3 minutes. Add the onions, vinegar and sesame oil and fry for 5 minutes, until the chicken is cooked. Transfer to a bowl. Stir-fry the cashews for 1 minute and sprinkle over the chicken. Serve with rice.

chicken

This popular meat is a power-pack of lean protein and a provider of B vitamins to give you a blast of sustained energy.

Lean meat is a top choice for anyone taking regular exercise, and organic chicken is one of the leanest, as long as you resist eating the skin. It provides a healthy dose of protein to build strength and keep bones strong, along with a pair of vitamins that maximize its energy value. Niacin and pyridoxine, or vitamins B3 and B6, work together to make the most of food's energizing potential. Chicken should always be bought organic: it is now widely available, and provides all the benefits without the risk of food-poisoning bacteria and drug residues.

NUTRIENTS
Vitamins B3, B6; phosphorus, selenium; protein; tryptophan

EASY CHICKEN MARINADE

3 tbsp soy sauce
3 tbsp rice wine or sherry
1 tsp sugar
2 cloves garlic, crushed
450g/1lb chicken breast, cut into bite-sized pieces

Mix together the soy sauce, wine, sugar and garlic. Place the chicken in a dish, pour over the marinade, cover and place in a cool place for 2 hours.

○ ⓒ ◉

cheese

Don't pass on the cheese: this nutritious food can build up your bones, and muscle strength, without adding anything to your weight.

Weight-bearing exercise builds strong bones, but it puts them under pressure, increasing the body's need for foods to build bone density. Famous for its high levels of calcium, cheese also contains phosphorus, which combines with calcium to strengthen the bones. It is also packed with protein, which builds muscle strength. Unfairly maligned as a high-fat food, cheese can be bought in a wide range of low-fat versions that are still nutritious. As with other products of animal origin, organic is best.

Eating cheese increases the body's ability to burn fat after a meal.

NUTRIENTS
Calcium, iodine, phosphorus, selenium; protein

WELSH RABBIT

4 slices bread
1 tbsp groundnut oil
150g/6oz Cheddar cheese, grated
1 tbsp brown ale
½ tsp mustard
black pepper to taste

Toast the bread under a grill. Heat the oil in a pan and add the cheese, ale and mustard. Stir over a gentle heat until thickened. Season with pepper and spoon over the toast. Put back under the grill until the cheese bubbles. Serve immediately.

NUTRIENTS
Vitamins B2, B5, B12, D, K;
iodine, molybdenum, phosphorus
selenium; protein

egg

Little capsules of strength and energy, eggs are rich in nutrients that will maximize your workout gains.

Eating the right meal within an hour or two after exercise could make the biggest difference you've noticed yet. That's the time when your body needs – and most effectively uses – food to turn your effort into stronger muscles and increased energy levels. It's also when you burn fat most effectively. Eggs are a concentrated source of muscle-building amino acids and other body-building nutrients. They're also rich in vitamin K, which helps to heal bruises and other minor sports injuries. This vitamin works by ensuring that blood is able to clot normally, so it could also reduce the danger of blood clots in arteries.

LEEK AND PEPPER OMELETTE

1 tbsp groundnut oil
1 leek, finely chopped
**1 sweet pepper, deseeded
    and diced**
4 eggs
salt and pepper to taste

Heat the oil and gently fry the leek for 2–3 minutes until half cooked.

Add the sweet pepper and cook for 2 minutes. Remove the vegetables with a slotted spoon and set aside. Beat the eggs in a bowl and add 2 tablespoons of cold water. Season and pour the mixture into the pan. Add the vegetables and cook for around 5 minutes until the egg is set.

tomato juice

Mineral-packed, this is the perfect post-workout drink and a healthy alternative to excessive water.

A tomato is packed with vitamins and minerals, but it is most renowned for the life-saving properties of a versatile phytonutrient called lycopene. Unusually, lycopene is unharmed by food processing, which means that tomato-based products offer many of the same benefits as the fresh fruit. A bottle of tomato juice keeps minerals at a safe level when you're running. Most of us get too much sodium in our diet, but a long run can dangerously reduce the body's levels of minerals, particularly sodium – especially if you've drunk a lot of water. A drink of bought tomato juice replenishes fluid and sodium.

NUTRIENTS

Vitamins A, B-complex, C, E, K, folate; chromium, copper, iron, magnesium, manganese, molybdenum, phosphorus, potassium; fibre; lycopene; protein

CHILLED TOMATO SOUP

8 tomatoes, skinned, deseeded and chopped
2 cucumbers, diced
1 litre/35fl oz/4 cups tomato juice
2 sweet peppers, deseeded and diced
2 cloves garlic, crushed
1 tbsp red wine vinegar

1 tbsp olive oil

Blend half the tomatoes, half the cucumber, the juice, sweet pepper, garlic and vinegar in a blender. Stir in the oil and remaining tomatoes and cucumber. Chill for 30 minutes before serving.

grapefruit

Eating a grapefruit at the start of a meal could help to stop you piling on the pounds.

Starting a meal with half a grapefruit is an old diet trick that does seem to work, according to scientists. In 2006, they found that this simple change helped a group of very overweight volunteers to lose weight. Their blood-sugar levels were healthier than usual afterwards, too. Other evidence suggests that eating grapefruit can steady insulin levels. So they could help to prevent the vicious cycle in which gaining weight leads to diabetes, and diabetes makes people put on even more weight. Grapefruit is full of flavonoids that repair cell damage, combat cancer and protect the heart.

NUTRIENTS
Vitamin C, beta carotene, folate; potassium; fibre; liminoids

A daily glass of grapefruit juice can significantly reduce the risk of kidney stones.

GRAPEFRUIT AND CHICKEN SALAD

2 grapefruits, unpeeled
4 tbsp honey vinaigrette (see page 29)
350g/12oz/2 cups cooked chicken, shredded
4 sweet peppers, deseeded and cut into rings

Grate the grapefruit zest and add to the vinaigrette. Pour over the chicken pieces. Peel the grapefruit and cut into wheels. Put the grapefruit wheels and the pepper rings into a dish and pile the chicken on top.

pear

Sweet and satisfying, pears are rich in fibre that helps the body shed excess weight.

Both soluble and insoluble fibre help to fill you up in a healthy way. Pears are among the few fruits that contain a high quantity of insoluble fibre, which gives them an enticing edge, both sweet and satisfying. Their sweet taste and refreshing juiciness make them an appealing option to anyone who has given up sugary treats in order to lose weight. Also, when people are trying to lose weight, the change in diet sometimes disturbs the eliminatory system. Pears counteract any tendency towards sluggish digestion if you're eating less than usual.

NUTRIENTS
Vitamin C; copper; fibre

GRILLED PEARS

4 ripe pears, halved and cored
2 tbsp currants
4 tbsp apple juice

Grill the pears under a low heat for about 5 minutes, turning once. Sprinkle the currants on top and pour over the apple juice. Serve immediately.

rock melon

NUTRIENTS
Vitamins B3, B6, C, beta carotene, folic acid; potassium; fibre

A mouth-watering slice of nutritional goodness that tops up your antioxidant levels too.

The dense texture of these fragrant melons makes them a satisfying replacement for the foods you're limiting, just as their sweetness meets the need otherwise filled by empty-calorie snacks. And a rock melon – also known as a cantaloupe or musk melon – contains more nutritional power than a plateful of bakery goods. Just one slice of melon provides more vitamin C and beta carotene than your body can use in a whole day. This kind of melon loses some of its vitamin C content quite quickly after cutting, so don't cut any more than the slice you're about to eat.

MELON AND GINGER

2 small rock melons
2 tsp lime juice
2.5cm/1in root ginger, finely chopped
2 tsp cinnamon
4 tbsp cherries (optional)

Quarter the melons and cut away the skin. Scoop out and discard the seeds. Cut into wedges or scoop into balls. Add the lime juice and ginger and mix together well. Dust with cinnamon, top with cherries, if using, and serve.

strawberry

This delicious and popular fruit contains a treasury of fat-fighting nutrition.

Strawberries are the sort of fruit people eat for pleasure, not in order to achieve their diet or health goals. So it's surprising to learn that they're packed with nutrients that aid weight control, along with many other healthy

A pinch of pepper adds a tasty edge to fresh strawberries.

effects. Their unusually rich supply of vitamins and minerals keeps energy levels high, reducing the urge to nibble. This delectable, bite-sized, finger-friendly fruit is a great replacement for sweets when you want a treat. And with more insoluble fibre than many other fruits, strawberries keep you fuller for longer.

NUTRIENTS
Vitamins B2, B5, B6, C, K, folic acid; copper, magnesium, manganese, iodine, potassium; anthocyanidins; flavonoids; fibre; omega-3 oils; ellagic acid

STRAWBERRY DELIGHT

4 mandarins
350g/12oz strawberries, dehulled
175g/6oz grapes
115g/4oz flaked almonds
2 tbsp orange juice (optional)

Divide the mandarins into segments. Place in a serving bowl and add the strawberries, grapes and almonds. Pour over the orange juice, if using, and mix well. Serve.

courgette

This energizing food makes salads more substantial and keeps blood sugar steady.

NUTRIENTS

Vitamins B1, B2, B6, C, K, beta carotene, folic acid; copper, magnesium, manganese, phosphorus, potassium; fibre

The numerous vitamins and minerals in courgettes, or zucchini, help to keep energy levels up while your food intake is down. It is particularly rich in manganese, which helps to regulate blood-sugar levels. Refined foods and sweet products make blood-sugar levels rise sharply, providing a quick burst of energy followed by a slump. Courgettes are high in fibre, which delays hunger pangs. They can be cooked in numerous ways or eaten raw as a snack or in salads.

Courgettes replace much of the beta carotene wiped out by smoking and drinking alcohol.

RATATOUILLE

2 aubergines, chopped into chunks
2 tbsp olive oil
2 onions, chopped
3 cloves garlic, crushed
4 courgettes, chopped
2 x 400g/14oz tin tomatoes

Sprinkle the aubergines with salt. Leave for 30 minutes, then rinse and dry. Heat the oil in a pan and fry the onions and aubergines for 5 minutes. Add the remaining ingredients, bring to the boil, and simmer for 10 minutes until the courgettes are cooked. Serve.

pea

These popular vegetables are little balls of nutrient energy, packed with fibre to keep hunger at bay.

Green, or English, peas are packed with all kinds of nutrients. They are exceptionally rich in fibre, one of nature's biggest aids to weight control. Scores of medical studies show that the more fibre you eat, the less likely you are to put on weight and the more readily you will lose it. By slowing down the rate at which food moves on from the stomach, it helps to keep blood-sugar and insulin levels steady. And it may also affect hormones in the intestine that control the appetite. Peas are rich in both soluble and insoluble fibre, helping to fill you up while keeping your digestive system healthy.

NUTRIENTS

Vitamins B-complex, C, K, beta carotene, folic acid; copper, iron, magnesium, manganese, phosphorus, potassium, zinc; fibre; protein

PEAS WITH MINT AND ORANGE

175g/6oz frozen petits pois
1 tsp grated orange zest
1 tbsp orange juice
1 tbsp chopped mint leaves
salt and pepper to taste

Bring a pan of water to the boil and add the peas and orange zest. Cook for 3 minutes until tender. Drain, add the orange juice and briefly heat. Stir in the mint leaves, season and serve.

garlic

NUTRIENTS

Vitamins B1, B6, C; calcium, copper, iron, manganese, phosphorus, potassium, selenium; protein

GARLIC SOUP

2 tbsp olive oil
4 cloves garlic, crushed
200g/7oz/2 cups fresh
 breadcrumbs
1 litre/35fl oz/4 cups hot
 vegetable stock
4 eggs (optional)

Heat the oil in a pan over a low heat and sauté the garlic for about 30 seconds. Add the breadcrumbs and sauté for 1 minute. Stir in the stock, bring to the boil, then simmer for 10 minutes. Break the eggs, if using, into the soup and poach for about 3 minutes. Serve with crusty bread.

Keeping weight down is just one of this wonder-working bulb's health-enhancing abilities.

Garlic is known for its powerful smell and taste, but its protective powers are even stronger, ranging from fighting cancer to promoting weight loss. Its strongest properties stem from a rich supply of compounds containing sulphur, which is what creates that distinctive smell.

After crushing garlic, wait 10 minutes before cooking it to increase the nutritional benefits.

Slimming aid

Allicin, a component of garlic, has been found to aid weight loss even if you make no other changes to your diet. At the same time, it lowers blood levels of insulin, reducing the risk of weight-related problems such as metabolic syndrome and diabetes. Garlic doesn't just discourage fat from clinging to your hips and thighs: even more importantly, it helps to prevent fatty deposits forming inside your arteries, where they gradually harden and restrict blood flow. People who are trying to lose weight often eat high-protein diets and take extra exercise. Both of these can set up an inflammatory response in the body, which can reduce resistance to disease. So add a clove of garlic a day to your diet, as it has been proved to counteract inflammation.

Taste the difference

Garlic helps to make low-calorie meals more tasty, providing added flavour with virtually no calories. Meanwhile, it also protects the heart, lowers blood pressure, combats numerous cancers and fights all kinds of infections.

GARLIC MUSHROOMS

2 tbsp olive oil
4 cloves garlic, crushed
450g/1lb mushrooms
4 slices wholemeal bread
(optional)

Heat the oil in a pan over a low heat and stir in the garlic. Add the mushrooms and cover with a tightly fitting lid. Cook over a very low heat for about 8 minutes, shaking occasionally, until the mushrooms are tender. Toast the bread, if using, pile the mushrooms on top and serve immediately.

rocket

This decorative little leaf is one of the most nutritious ingredients you can find in a salad.

NUTRIENTS

Vitamins B-complex, C, K, beta carotene, folic acid; calcium, iron, magnesium, manganese, phosphorus, potassium, zinc; fibre

TRIPLE-TASTE SALAD

12 Webbs lettuce leaves
115g/4oz rocket leaves
115g/4oz curly endive or
raddichio
1 tbsp walnut oil
1 tbsp vinegar

Tear the lettuce leaves and mix together with the rocket and curly endive. Mix together the walnut oil and vinegar and pour over just before serving.

Salad is an ideal low-calorie meal, not least because the raw ingredients encourage you to eat slowly. This gives the body time to register when you've had enough, instead of 10 minutes later, which can happen if you eat quickly. The peppery taste of rocket (also known as arugula, rucola or roquette) livens up a leaf-based salad. The vitamins and minerals it contains work together to preserve bone health – a concern if you've cut down on calcium-rich dairy foods while trying to lose weight.

One serving of rocket provides more than the daily requirement of bone-building vitamin K.

chilli

These fiery hot peppers could burn away some unwanted weight as they raise your temperature.

Some experts say that chillies increase the body's fat-burning ability for about 20 minutes after a meal, so that you are literally burning up the food you've just eaten faster than normal. Others say that the fiery taste simply makes you eat more slowly, or that the tastiness makes food more satisfying. Whatever the reason, adding some of these hot peppers to your everyday diet does seem to aid weight control. They also alleviate chronic indigestion and kill the bacteria that cause stomach ulcers, though eating too many could lead to stomach cancer.

NUTRIENTS
Vitamin C, beta carotene; iron, potassium; fibre

ROAST CHILLI RELISH

200g/7oz fresh chillies, deseeded
1 tbsp olive oil
4 cloves garlic, crushed
1 cucumber, finely chopped

Grill the chillies for 4–5 minutes until the skins blister. Put in a sealed plastic bag for 10 minutes. Rub the skins off and finely chop the chillies. Mix with the remaining ingredients. Keep in the fridge for up to 2 weeks. Use sparingly.

060

almond

The ideal replacement for an empty-calorie snack, almonds will keep you going for longer.

Almonds may seem an odd weight-loss choice because they contain quite a lot of fat. But when scientists put two groups of people on low-calorie diets, one of which included almonds, the almond-eating group lost 50 per cent more weight and fat than the others. Almonds are rich in monounsaturated fat, which helps you feel fuller for longer, and their high fibre content helps to keep blood-sugar levels steady and prevent hunger pangs. A dozen almonds contains just 90 calories along with a burst of protein and nutrients that combine to increase energy levels.

NUTRIENTS
Vitamins B2, E; copper, magnesium, manganese, phosphorus; protein

ALMOND SALSA

2 tbsp almonds
2 tomatoes, chopped
2 red onions, finely diced
2 tbsp finely cut chives
1 tbsp chopped parsley
2 tsp vinegar

Dry-fry the almonds briefly in a frying pan. Mix together the tomatoes, onions, chives, parsley and vinegar in a bowl. Add the almonds and serve.

rye

This high-fibre, low-GI cereal star aids weight loss and combats fluid retention.

Wholegrain cereals play an important role in weight loss. Full of insoluble fibre, they score low on the glycaemic index (GI), meaning they release sugar into the blood slowly, whereas refined versions have little nutritional value and cause a sudden spike in energy, then a slump. Low-GI foods have long been known to benefit health, but they have now also proved to aid fat loss, even when you eat the same number of calories as on a higher-GI diet. Rye is one of the lowest GI cereals. It's also rich in compounds that bind to water from food, which prevents bloating.

NUTRIENTS

Magnesium, phosphorus, selenium; lignans; fibre; protein

COTTAGE CHEESE ON RYE

8 slices rye bread
8 tbsp cottage cheese
1 tsp finely sliced lemongrass
4 tomatoes, roughly chopped
4 gherkins, sliced

Toast the bread. Mix together the cottage cheese and lemongrass. Pile onto the toast and top with the tomatoes and gherkins. Serve immediately.

062

tofu

NUTRIENTS

Calcium, copper, iron, magnesium, manganese, phosphorus, potassium; fibre; omega-3 oils; protein; tryptophan

The wonder-working soy bean could protect your organs while smoothing your silhouette.

Best known for its beneficial effects on women's hormones, tofu, or bean curd, may also help to maintain a healthy weight for both sexes. It's made from fermented soy beans. Among soy's many healthy components is an isoflavone called genistein, which seems to promote fat loss by reducing the size and number of fat cells. Women using soy bean to treat menopausal symptoms have found that it also prevented weight gain, especially on the abdomen – a common effect of the changes in hormone levels after the menstrual cycle stops.

TOFU SKEWERS

4 tbsp soy sauce
1 tbsp sesame oil
1 tbsp sweet apple juice
pinch of chilli powder
450g/1lb firm tofu, drained and cubed
4 sweet peppers, deseeded and chopped into chunks

Mix together the soy sauce, sesame oil, apple juice and chilli powder and use to marinate the tofu for at least an hour. Thread the tofu and peppers alternately onto skewers. Grill or bake for 5–10 minutes until brown, basting often with the remaining marinade. Serve.

TOFU SMOOTHIE

200g/7oz tofu
8 tbsp orange juice
8 tbsp mango pulp
4 apples, chopped
4 tbsp chopped walnuts

Put all the ingredients except for 1 tablespoon of the walnuts into a blender. Blend on a low speed until the ingredients are mixed, then on a high speed until the mixture is smooth. Pour into glasses, top with the remaining walnuts, and serve.

Get the balance right

Soy reduces the risk of many diseases: cancers, heart disease, osteoporosis and diabetes, but its powerful effects on hormones could stimulate hormone-dependent cancers or thyroid problems, so it should not be overused. Traditional Asian foods such as tofu, miso and natto are the healthiest option; the long-term effects of new products are not known.

Soy's healthy effects are stronger in tofu than in other soy products.

tuna

This is a low-fat, high-protein food with a secret ingredient to aid weight control.

Popular sources of protein, such as meat products and hard cheese, are often high in fat. Yet high-protein foods keep you going longer before flagging energy levels send you in search of a snack. Tuna is an excellent low-fat option. It's one of the richest sources of protein, providing more than even the healthiest meat. The best choices are albacore, skipjack or yellowfin tuna. And fresh tuna is rich in omega-3 oils. Among its many other benefits, omega-3 stimulates production of a hormone called leptin that controls the appetite.

NUTRIENTS
Vitamins B1, B3, B6; magnesium, phosphorus, potassium, selenium; omega-3 oils; protein; tryptophan

BAKED TUNA

4 fresh tuna steaks
black pepper to taste
3 tbsp olive oil
2 onions, chopped
8 tbsp dry white wine
4 tomatoes, chopped

Preheat the oven to 220°C/ 425°F/Gas 7. Put the tuna in a baking dish and rub with the pepper and 1 tablespoon of the oil. Heat the remaining oil in a frying pan and sauté the onions for 3–5 minutes. Add the wine and tomatoes, and bring to the boil. Pour over the tuna and bake for 15 minutes, until the tuna is cooked through. Serve.

cottage cheese

Rich in protein and calcium, this has all you want from dairy food without the high fat content.

Dairy foods are sometimes shunned because they're seen as laden with saturated fat, but they may help in losing weight. Some studies have found that a high-calcium diet decreases the body's absorption of fat, possibly causing it to be burnt off faster. A 100g/3½oz serving of low-fat cottage cheese contains more than 60mg calcium for only 1–4g fat (hard cheese contains more calcium, but up to a third of its weight is fat). Cottage cheese is also rich in protein and the bone-building minerals that may be lacking in a low-dairy diet.

Try cottage cheese with pepper as a low-fat replacement for mayonnaise.

NUTRIENTS
Vitamins B2, B12; calcium, iodine, phosphorus, selenium; protein

COTTAGE CHEESE AND VEGETABLE SALAD

175g/6oz green beans, chopped
4 small courgettes, grated
1 tbsp lemon juice
350g/12oz cottage cheese
4 tbsp sunflower seeds

Steam the green beans for 5 minutes until tender. Mix together with the courgettes and lemon juice. Top with the cottage cheese, sprinkle over the seeds and serve.

065

○ ◑ ✦ ♡ ➖

cider vinegar

Use this vinegar to make food seem more filling
and keep hunger at bay for longer afterwards.

NUTRIENTS
Vitamin C; manganese, potassium;
acetic acid; pectin

Taking a few drops of vinegar with or before a meal has been
proved to help people lose weight. Cider vinegar, which is rich
in nutrients, has the added benefit of reducing the indigestion
that can accompany a change in diet. This can cause pangs
that feel like hunger even when you've just eaten. Vinegar's
acetic acid content makes you feel full up sooner and for
longer. This feeling of satiety stems from a reduction
in the glycaemic index (GI) of the food you eat. Foods
with a high GI (including most highly processed items)
go through your system quickly, leaving you ready for
more. Vinegar reduces the GI and lets food stay longer in
your stomach. It also reduces the risk of a mid-afternoon
energy slump sending you in search of a snack.

CREAMY SALAD DRESSING

2 tbsp cider vinegar
2 tsp apple juice
4 tbsp low-fat yogurt
1 clove garlic, crushed
1 tsp chopped thyme

Place all the ingredients in a
bowl and whisk together. Chill
and serve the dressing on your
favourite salad.

green tea

This health-giving drink could reduce weight while protecting you from a wide range of diseases.

NUTRIENTS
A wide range of polyphenols

Don't drink green tea in early pregnancy as it may increase the risk of spina bifida.

Few foods excite scientists as much as green tea, with its phenomenal range of health benefits. It also plays a dual role in helping you shape up: firstly by increasing exercise endurance and secondly by inhibiting the action of enzymes that help turn food into fat, especially around the midriff, where stored fat increases the risk of heart disease and diabetes. You can reap its benefits from 3–4 cups a day. Use boiling water for the full health benefits, or slightly cooler water for a less bitter taste.

GREEN TEA REFRESHER

6 tsp green tea leaves
500ml/18fl oz/2 cups apple or peach juice
4 tsp runny honey (optional)

Pour 250ml/9fl oz/1 cup boiled water onto the tea leaves. Brew for 3–5 minutes, strain into a jug and leave to cool. Stir in the juice and honey, then pour over ice into glasses and serve.

apricot

Life is sweet: this juicy fruit tastes good and helps you feel good too.

Just as popular fresh or dried, apricots are rich in the amino acid tryptophan, which the body converts to the feel-good chemical serotonin. This brain chemical lifts your mood, making you feel more optimistic, improving self-esteem and even helping to control impulsive behaviour. And it helps you sleep well too. Some of the tryptophan is also converted to niacin, or vitamin B3, if necessary. A shortage of this can cause lethargy, so eating apricots can keep energy levels high.

NUTRIENTS

Vitamins A, C; carotenoids; fibre; potassium; tryptophan

APRICOT AND RICOTTA TREATS

4 tbsp ricotta cheese
2 tsp honey
8 ripe apricots, halved and stoned
8 almond halves

Mix the ricotta with the honey and fill the apricots with the mixture. Stud the apricots with the almond halves and serve.

◎ ◐ ♥ ⓒ ◉ ≡

banana

A classic comfort food that cheers you up without the after-effects of a junk-food binge.

A banana is often a favourite fruit of babies and children and in adult life can trigger feelings of being safe and nurtured. Rich in healthy carbohydrates, they're ideal when you crave comfort foods, as they feel enjoyably self-indulgent and they're stuffed with nutrients that soothe and lift your mood. A great source of vitamin B6, bananas reduce fatigue and premenstrual symptoms. They also contain potassium, to relieve irritability, and tryptophan, to ease depression and promote healthy sleep.

NUTRIENTS
Vitamins B6, C; manganese; potassium; fibre; tryptophan

GRILLED BANANAS

4 bananas, peeled
4 tsp lemon juice
2 tsp cinnamon
2 tbsp almonds

Slice the bananas in half lengthways and place on an oiled baking sheet. Sprinkle with the lemon juice and cinnamon and place under a hot grill until the bananas start to brown. Scatter the almonds over, and serve.

asparagus

These slender spears are forceful weapons against lethargy and low spirits.

Give yourself a natural high by eating asparagus. They taste delicious and supply numerous minerals and vitamins, including many of the B vitamins, which play a central role in supporting brain function and the nervous system. If any of these are in short supply you may be tired, depressed, anxious or constantly on edge. This can happen quite easily if you're not eating a wide range of healthy foods. B vitamins work best together, rather than individually, keeping energy levels high and supporting mental and emotional health.

NUTRIENTS
Vitamins A, B-complex, C, K, folic acid; copper, manganese, phosphorus, potassium; fibre; protein

ASPARAGUS WITH HONEY AND GARLIC

450g/1lb asparagus
1 tsp mustard
2 tbsp runny honey
2 cloves garlic, crushed
½ tsp chopped thyme leaves

Steam the asparagus for 5 minutes until just tender. Drain and put on a plate. Mix together the mustard, honey, garlic and thyme, and pour over the asparagus. Serve immediately.

avocado

This creamy fruit provides healthy fats, which raise serotonin levels and keep you happy.

A low-fat diet really can get you down! Scientists have found that people are more relaxed after a higher-fat meal, and even feel less pain. Some fat is also necessary for the body to absorb nutrients that can improve your mood, such as vitamin E. No wonder people eat junk foods when they're feeling low. Avocados are the healthier alternative: instead of saturated fat, they provide healthy monounsaturated fat. They are rich in tryptophan, along with vitamin B6 and folic acid, which helps the body turn tryptophan into the feel-good chemical serotonin.

NUTRIENTS
Vitamins B6, C, K, folic acid; copper, potassium; carotenoids; fibre; monounsaturated fats; tryptophan

AVOCADO WITH PAPRIKA

4 ripe avocados, halved and
  stoned
2 tsp paprika
2 tsp lemon juice
4 slices wholemeal toast

Remove the avocado flesh from the skins and mash with a fork. Add the paprika and lemon juice and mix well. Serve spread on wholemeal toast.

sea vegetables

NUTRIENTS

Vitamins B2, B5, K, folic acid; calcium, iodine, iron, magnesium; lignans

---

LAVER CAKES

450g/1lb laver, or rehydrated cooked nori, chopped
225g/8oz/1¾ cups oatmeal
1 tsp ground black pepper
3 tbsp oil
450g/1lb portobello mushrooms

Mix together the laver, oatmeal and pepper in a bowl. Using your hands, shape into 12 balls and flatten slightly to make cakes. Heat 2 tablespoons of the oil and fry the cakes for 2–3 minutes. Brush the mushrooms with the remaining oil and grill. Serve together.

These gifts from the ocean could help to soothe away stress and put an end to insomnia by promoting peaceful sleep.

Look out for different forms of sea vegetables, such as laver (nori), wakame, dulse and others.

Sea vegetables or seaweeds, best known for their use in Japanese cuisine, contain an unrivalled range of nutrients that promote emotional health and keep the brain alert. They contain a wide range of minerals: magnesium helps to relieve stress-related symptoms such as heart palpitations; calcium helps to stabilize moods; and iron provides energy to the many people – especially young women – whose iron stores are low. The wide range of sea vegetables now available are rich in iodine, which supports thyroid function. A slightly underactive thyroid, which is fairly common, especially among women, often causes depression and lethargy before any other signs lead to diagnosis.

Helping hormones

Seaweed is among the foods credited with helping Japanese women keep their legendary composure through life's changes. Seaweed contains phytonutrients called lignans, which work as a gentle form of hormone-replacement therapy. Eaten regularly, they could help to reduce stress-inducing symptoms of the perimenopause, such as hot flushes. The plentiful nutrients found in sea vegetables could also relieve sleeplessness. The calming effects of magnesium, in particular, may counteract insomnia. Along with calcium, it can also prevent the leg cramps and restlessness that keep many women awake at night after the menopause.

MISO SOUP

4 tbsp chopped dulse
2 tbsp wakame
2.5cm/1in root ginger, finely
   chopped
115g/4oz tofu, cut into cubes
3 tbsp miso

Pour 1.2litres/44fl oz/5 cups of water into a pan and add the seaweeds, ginger and tofu. Bring to the boil and simmer for 5 minutes. Stir in the miso, heat for 2 minutes and serve.

sweet potato

When you're feeling low and longing for a sweet treat, this will give your mood a healthy lift.

How can something that provides all the comfort of sweetness and carbohydrates be good for you? Easy, when it's a sweet potato. This cheery tuber is packed with nutrients that help to raise your spirits. It is rich in iron, so can offset any deficiency, especially for women during their periods, and in vitamin B6. This vital vitamin alleviates premenstrual syndrome and food cravings, as well as helping to relieve depression. It also keeps blood-sugar levels steady, helping to prevent mood swings.

NUTRIENTS

Vitamins B6, C, beta carotene; copper, iron, potassium; fibre

BAKED SWEET POTATOES

4 sweet potatoes, unpeeled
225g/8oz cottage cheese
2 tbsp chopped chives
2 tsp chopped coriander
2 tsp paprika
salt and pepper to taste

Pierce the skin of the potatoes 4 times. Bake in an oven at 200°C/400°F/Gas 6 for 1 hour until soft inside. Mix together the remaining ingredients. Cut the potatoes open and scoop out the flesh. Mix with the other ingredients and put back into the skins. Season to taste and serve immediately.

○ ◑ ◖ ♡

cinnamon

This revitalizing spice could sharpen up your cognitive abilities and counteract mood swings.

Cinnamon has a surprisingly strong effect on the brain and moods, scientists have found. Its distinctive smell works directly on the brain to increase alertness. It has been found to help students concentrate more effectively in exams, and may slow down the onset of cognitive decline in old age. Through a different process, cinnamon can help to prevent mood swings caused by fluctuating blood-sugar levels. And as little as half a teaspoonful a day could help to control diabetes.

NUTRIENTS
Calcium, iron, manganese; fibre

CINNAMON POACHED FRUIT

250ml/9fl oz/1 cup white wine
zest and juice of ½ lemon
2 tbsp cinnamon
4 pears, cored and chopped
8 apricots, stoned and chopped
4 tbsp chopped dried fruit of choice

Place the wine, lemon juice, zest and cinnamon into a large pan. Bring to the boil. Add the fruit and return to the boil. Reduce the heat and simmer for 2 minutes. Leave to stand for at least 10 minutes. Serve with yogurt, ricotta cheese or ice cream.

rosemary

Rosemary is for remembrance: its evocative fragrance can help to keep your memories fresh.

Rosemary has traditionally been prized for its ability to improve the memory, and it's not a myth: this herb can help to counteract a tendency to forgetfulness. A compound called rosmarinic acid improves blood circulation, increasing the flow of oxygen-rich blood to the brain. This improves all kinds of brain functions, aiding concentration and alertness. People perform better in memory tests, and have been found to be more alert, when they work in a room smelling of rosemary. And at the same time they also feel more relaxed and contented.

NUTRIENTS

Calcium, iron, manganese; bioflavonoids; fibre

ROSEMARY POTATOES

450g/1lb potatoes, cut
   into wedges
2 tbsp groundnut oil
1 clove garlic, crushed
   (optional)
black pepper to taste
1 tbsp chopped fresh rosemary

Boil the potato wedges for 10 minutes until tender. Heat the oil and sauté the garlic and potatoes until the potatoes are browned and crunchy. Add the pepper and rosemary for the final minute of cooking time and serve immediately.

⊚ ⟿ ⊙ ⟆ ⟆ ⊚

sage

This fragrant herb is a wise choice to keep you mentally alert, comfortably cool and sleeping well.

NUTRIENTS
Calcium, iron; polyphenols

Sage has several ways of improving mind and mood. It has been proved in research to increase brain power, particularly short-term memory, as in word-recall tests. It contains compounds similar to drugs that are used to combat the formation of plaques in the brain, and research is now under way to find out if it can slow the progression of Alzheimer's disease. Sage can also ease the symptoms of the perimenopause. By preventing hot flushes and night sweats, it promotes healthy sleep patterns.

Sprinkle a handful of roughly torn sage leaves onto a salad to make it even more nutritious.

SQUASH SOUP WITH SAGE

450g/1lb deseeded and chopped squash
500ml/18fl oz/2 cups stock
1 tbsp oil
2 onions, chopped
4 tbsp chopped sage leaves
black pepper to taste

Boil the squash for 10 minutes until tender. Place in a blender, add the stock and purée until smooth. Heat the oil in a large pan. Sauté the onions for 3 minutes and add half the sage for the last minute. Add the squash mixture and bring to the boil. Simmer for 10 minutes, stir in the pepper and the remaining sage, and serve.

kidney bean

This small but powerful food provides an armoury of nutrients to keep you on top form.

The humble kidney bean provides an impressive array of nutrients for combating low moods and strengthening brain function. Rich in vitamin B1, it keeps the memory sharp and its rich magnesium content promotes physical and mental relaxation. The soluble fibre keeps blood-sugar levels steady, giving you plenty of vitality while preventing energy spikes and slumps, and it provides a mineral top-up for the many women whose periods leave them short of iron. On top of that, the high protein content helps to keep your strength up.

NUTRIENTS

Vitamins B1, K, folic acid; copper, iron, magnesium, manganese, molybdenum, phosphorus, potassium; fibre; protein

CHILLI BEANS

1 tbsp groundnut oil
2 onions, chopped
1 tsp chilli powder or 1 fresh chilli, chopped
225g/8oz lean minced beef (optional)
400g/14oz tin kidney beans, drained
400g/14oz tin tomatoes

Heat the oil in a pan and fry the onions for 2–3 minutes. Add the chilli and fry for another minute. Stir in the beef, if using, and cook until browned. Add the beans and tomatoes and bring to the boil. Reduce the heat and simmer for 10 minutes. Serve with brown rice.

brown rice

A versatile grain that eases stress at all ages and smooths the path through the perimenopause.

Many of the nutrients that could improve mood more effectively are lost when rice is processed to become white. Brown rice still contains all its nutrients and provides selenium, which counters depression but is lacking in most people's diets. It's also rich in magnesium, which plays a major role in reducing mood swings and easing stress. Brown rice takes longer than white varieties to digest, preventing a sudden rise and fall in blood-sugar levels and making you feel comfortably full. Packed with phytonutrients, it is particularly useful in countering mood swings and other symptoms of the perimenopause.

NUTRIENTS
Magnesium, manganese, selenium; fibre; tryptophan

RICE PUDDING

300g/10oz/1½ cups brown rice
4 tbsp raisins
250ml/9fl oz/1 cup milk
2 tbsp runny honey
2 tsp cinnamon

Boil the rice for 15 minutes, until tender. Preheat the oven to 160°C/ 325°F/Gas 3. Mix together the rice and raisins in a baking dish. In a pan, gently heat the milk and honey. Pour over the rice and sprinkle with cinnamon. Bake for 30 minutes and serve.

brazil nut

This tasty snack contains a rare source of a mineral that can protect against depression and anxiety.

Could a few nuts really be the answer to depression, for some people? Brazil nuts are the richest source of a mood-boosting mineral called selenium. People whose diets are deficient in this have been found to suffer depression, anxiety and fatigue, and to feel better when they eat selenium-rich food. In much of the world even a healthy diet may be low in selenium, because foods are often grown in depleted soil. The harmless Brazil nut contains other mood-enhancing nutrients too, such as magnesium, which soothes stress and anxiety. Just a couple of brazil nuts are enough to meet most people's selenium levels.

NUTRIENTS
Vitamin B1; copper, magnesium, manganese, phosphorus, selenium; fibre; protein

HAPPY SALAD

225g/8oz salad potatoes, halved
250g/8oz baby spinach leaves
4 small sweet peppers, deseeded and chopped
salad dressing to taste
115g/4oz/¾ cup Brazil nuts, chopped
1 tbsp sunflower seeds

Boil the potatoes for 10 minutes, until tender. Put in a bowl and add the spinach and peppers. Mix together the nuts and seeds. Pour over the dressing, pile the nuts and seeds on top and serve.

sunflower seed

Combat fatigue, ease tension and keep the brain working well by munching on this healthy snack.

People who are busy and stressed tend to eat badly when they most need good nutrition. Seeds of all kinds are nutritious, and easy to eat on the run; the sunflower variety is among the best sources of nutrients that support mental and emotional health. They are rich in vitamin E, which may reduce the risk of Alzheimer's and prevent stressful hot flushes. Vitamin E and magnesium also combat insomnia. They are also rich in the B vitamins, which are central to our psychological well-being. B1, in particular, helps to keep the brain alert under stress.

Sunflower seeds are also among the richest sources of phytosterols, which can reduce cholesterol.

NUTRIENTS
Vitamins B1, B5, E, folic acid; copper, magnesium, manganese, phosphorus, selenium

SUNFLOWER TOPPING

1 tbsp groundnut oil
4 tbsp sunflower seeds
1 tbsp sesame seeds
2 tbsp walnut halves
1 tbsp soy sauce
2.5cm/1in root ginger, finely chopped

Heat the oil in a wok until very hot, throw in the seeds and walnuts and fry for 30 seconds, stirring all the time. Add the soy sauce and transfer to a bowl immediately. Add the ginger. Serve sprinkled on rice or stir-fries.

linseed

NUTRIENTS
Vitamin B6, folic acid; copper, magnesium, manganese, phosphorus; fibre; lignans; omega-3 oils

BREAKFAST BOOST

4 tbsp linseed
2 bananas, sliced
½ small rock melon, deseeded and chopped
4 tsp pumpkin seeds
2 tsp sesame seeds
8 tbsp low-fat yogurt
115g/4oz strawberries, dehulled and chopped

Place the ingredients, except for the strawberries, in a bowl and mix together well. Serve topped with the strawberries.

This tiny wonder-food, also known as flax seed, can lift depression, aid concentration, increase energy levels and smooth out hormonal changes.

Whatever your age or sex, linseed could make you feel happier and help you to think more clearly. This superseed contains nutrients that are vital to brain functioning, but are lacking in most people's diets. For women aged over 35, it can also alleviate stressful perimenopausal symptoms such as hot flushes, insomnia and mood swings. It also keeps the body's production of hormones and other chemicals in balance. This prevents hormonal upheaval caused by premenstrual syndrome or a malfunctioning thyroid.

Linseed is rich in compounds called lignans, which the body converts into hormone-like substances that smooth out fluctuating hormone levels. It is also one of the richest sources of omega-3 essential fatty acids, renowned for their benefits to mind and body.

One of the ways omega-3 helps to keep the brain and nervous system working smoothly is by allowing cells to function and communicate with each other properly. This can prevent many disorders that we think of as psychological. It also increases mental alertness and memory.

Getting the benefits

Linseed contains a form of omega-3 called alpha linolenic acid (ALA), but our ability to use it is reduced by saturated and hydrogenated fats, which compete for the same receptors in our bodies. So cut down on these fats and eat foods rich in vitamins B3, B6 and C, plus zinc and magnesium, which help the body to absorb ALA. Linseed oil is rich in omega-3, but does not contain lignans and loses much of its value if used in cooking.

1 tbsp linseed contains nearly all the omega-3 you need in a day.

oyster

NUTRIENTS
Vitamins A, B-complex, D, E; calcium, copper, iodine, iron, potassium, selenium, zinc; omega-3 oils

A dozen fresh oysters contains only about 110 calories.

Famed for putting a sparkle back in your sex life, these molluscs are also packed with omega-3.

Oysters are renowned for being an aphrodisiac, restoring libido to people who don't enjoy sex any more. That's partly because they're so rich in zinc, along with practically all the other minerals we need for good health. When the body is short of vital nutrients, sex is low on the list of functions it needs to maintain. Packed with nutrients, oysters act as a general health tonic as well as enhancing sexual well-being. They are a very rich, low-fat source of omega-3 fatty acids, which make us feel happier and livelier by supporting the brain's healthy functioning. They are also full of B vitamins, essential to mind and mood.

GREEN OYSTERS

24 fresh oysters
450g/1lb fresh spinach, chopped
115g/4oz fresh parsley, chopped
4 tbsp white wine

Preheat the oven to 220°C/425°F/ Gas 7. Open the oysters, remove from the shells and wash, discarding any already open. Place on half shells in a baking dish. Mix together the spinach, parsley and white wine. Spread over the oysters and bake for 6–7 minutes, until cooked through, and serve.

milk

Stay calm but alert with a drink that can combat premenstrual symptoms.

Many women become irritable, forgetful or depressed before a period starts – the well-known symptoms of premenstrual syndrome (PMS). A glass of milk could be the simplest answer, as it contains many nutrients that lift and stabilize mood. It's rich in calcium and vitamin D, which together have been found to reduce or even prevent PMS symptoms. As with other animal foods, it's best to buy organic. Organic milk has been found to contain up to 70 per cent more omega-3 oils, which help the brain to function. Have cold milk when you need to stay awake: it triggers the brain's production of dopamine and noradrenaline, which keep you alert.

NUTRIENTS
Vitamins A, B2, B12, D, K; calcium, iodine, phosphorus, potassium; protein

CEREAL SOOTHER

350g/12oz wholegrain breakfast cereal
4 tbsp sunflower seeds
2 bananas, sliced
250ml/9fl oz/1 cup skimmed or semi-skimmed milk

Mix together the cereal and the seeds in a large serving bowl. Serve topped with the banana and the milk poured over.

blueberry

This sometimes tart little fruit is a powerful weapon in the fight against age-related damage.

NUTRIENTS
Vitamins C, E; manganese; fibre

When researchers compile a list of the best foods for fighting free-radical cell damage, blueberries are usually in the top 10. Their colour comes from anthocyanins, which are believed to combat cell damage. They contain tannin, which combats inflammation, and resveratrol, a compound that fights cancer and heart disease. A diet rich in berries has been found to protect against dementia and preserve memory and learning ability in old age. Blueberries can also help prevent urinary tract infection and keep vision clear and may help to reverse neurodegenerative symptoms such as loss of balance and co-ordination.

BLUEBERRY AND PEAR CRUMBLE

85g/3oz butter
85g/3oz/¾ cup plain flour
40g/1½oz/½ cup porridge oats
4 tbsp brown sugar
2 large pears, cored and sliced
4 tbsp blueberries

Preheat the oven to 180°C/350°F/Gas 4. Rub the butter into the flour and porridge oats in a mixing bowl until the mixture is like breadcrumbs. Stir in the brown sugar. Mix together the pears and blueberries in a greased baking dish. Sprinkle the crumble mixture over the top and cook for 40–45 minutes until browned on top.

⊚♡ⓒ👁

fig

A tasty fruit that contains minerals to keep bones strong, and helps a sluggish digestive system.

NUTRIENTS
Beta carotene; calcium, manganese; potassium; fibre

> **Fig leaves, which can also be eaten, contain compounds that lower blood fats and combat diabetes.**

Two of the minerals in figs help to protect our bones: calcium, whose value is well known, and potassium. Most of us eat too much sodium (mainly from salt) and not enough potassium, which balances some of sodium's effects. While excess sodium causes the body to excrete calcium, potassium helps to reduce this loss. It also counteracts sodium's harmful effects on blood pressure. Figs' other main value is in relieving constipation, which is often a problem in later life. A compote made with rehydrated dried figs can cure it effectively.

SPICED FIGS

12 dried figs, soaked overnight
2 tbsp raisins
125ml/4fl oz/½ cup red wine
½ tsp ground cloves
2 tsp cinnamon
pinch of black pepper

Drain the figs, reserving 2 tablespoons of the water. Blend together with all the ingredients in a blender. Place in a saucepan, and gently heat for 5 minutes. Serve topped with ricotta cheese or yogurt.

cherry

NUTRIENTS

Vitamins B-complex, C; calcium, potassium; ellagic acid; flavonoids; fibre

Bones and joints feel the benefit of this juicy treat, which may even hold the key to staying young.

Aching joints and fragile bones are an unwelcome symptom of ageing, but cherries can do a lot to protect them. Their rich anthocyanin content acts as a powerful anti-inflammatory, combating pain in joints and muscles. This has the added benefit of helping people to stay active, which promotes general good health as well as bone strength and physical coordination. And it is the anthocyanins in cherries that give them the same heart-protective effects as red wine.

Another way in which cherries help is by supplying the mineral boron, which may help to prevent the steady loss of bone density with advancing age.

CHERRY SALAD

1 head of cos or romaine lettuce
450g/1lb cherries, stoned
2 ripe pears or apples, cored and chopped
115g/4oz cheese, cubed
salad dressing to taste
55g/2oz walnut halves

Tear the lettuce leaves and mix together with the fruit and cheese in a bowl. Pour the salad dressing over, top with the walnut halves and serve.

CHERRY HOT-OR-COLD SOUP

450g/1lb cherries, stoned
1 tsp cinnamon
zest and juice of ½ lemon
4 tbsp red wine
4 tbsp honey

Blend the cherries, cinnamon and lemon with 125ml/4fl oz/½ cup water. Pour into a saucepan and add the wine and honey. Heat gently over a low heat for about 5 minutes. Serve hot or chilled and top with yogurt, if wished.

Sweet (and sour) dreams

Sleeplessness often comes with later age, and cherries may help there, too. They contain melatonin, the nutrient that plays an important role in promoting healthy sleep patterns; it's often used to combat jetlag. Sour cherries are even richer in melatonin than their sweet relatives. On top of all that, cherries are rich in a number of flavonoids that protect the heart and reduce the risk of cancer.

The antioxidant effects of cherries are stronger than those of most other foods.

○ ✋ ⟨⟩ ♥ ⓒ 👁 ⬤

pomegranate

NUTRIENTS
Vitamin C, beta carotene, folic acid; potassium; ellagic acid; fibre

An ancient symbol of life and good luck that keeps its promise in later age.

Drinking a glass of pomegranate juice a day could help to protect you against three major problems of old age: heart disease, cancer and osteoarthritis. In men who already have prostate cancer, pomegranate has been found to slow the rate at which tumours grow. It may also reduce the risk of developing various cancers. The pomegranate's abundant polyphenols work as powerful antioxidants, preventing heart damage and build-up of plaque in the arteries. It can ease the pain and disability of osteoarthritis by slowing the deterioration of cartilage in the joints and preventing inflammation.

POMEGRANATE CREAM

200ml/7fl oz/¾ cup yogurt
2 tsp honey
4 ripe pomegranates
4 sprigs mint

Place the yogurt in a small bowl and stir in the honey until well combined. Cut each pomegranate in half horizontally and, using a wooden spoon, bash until the seeds fall out. Mix the pomegranate seeds with the yogurt and honey mixture, garnish with mint, and serve.

aubergine

The polished purple skin of this plant has very powerful and protective qualities.

Some people need more iron in their diet, but too much iron isn't a good thing. It increases the body's production of free radicals, byproducts of metabolic processes that damage the cells. Aubergines contain a host of phytonutrients that mop up harmful free radicals. One of them is chlorogenic acid, a powerful antioxidant that lowers levels of harmful cholesterol and has antibacterial and antiviral properties. Another is nasunin, which can also help the body excrete excess iron. This reduces the risk of conditions such as cancer, heart disease and arthritis.

NUTRIENTS
Vitamins B1, B3, B6, folate; copper, magnesium, manganese, potassium

BABA GANNOUSH

2 large aubergines
6 cloves garlic, crushed
4 tbsp tahini
4 tbsp lemon juice
1 tbsp olive oil
bunch of parsley

Preheat the oven to 190°C/375°F/Gas 5. Bake the aubergines on a baking tray for 30 minutes. Slice in half, scoop out and chop the insides. Leave in a colander to drain for at least 10 minutes. In a bowl, mash the aubergine with the garlic, tahini and lemon juice until a smooth paste. Pour olive oil over, and sprinkle with parsley. Serve with bread and crudités.

○ ○ ○ ○ ○ ○ ○ ○

cabbage

One plant carries a whole arsenal of weapons to defend against cancers and Alzheimer's.

NUTRIENTS
Vitamins A, B1, B2, B6, C, K, folate; calcium, magnesium, manganese, potassium; fibre; omega-3 oils; protein

As a cruciferous vegetable, cabbage fights cancer on many fronts. Its various compounds help the liver remove toxins, stop cells proliferating and prevent oestrogen from stimulating the growth of breast cancers. It also combats arthritis and eye disease. Red cabbage is richest in vitamin C and cancer-protective phytonutrients and can protect against Alzheimer's. Its anthocyanins counteract the effects of a chemical called beta-amyloid protein, which can damage brain cells. Let cruciferous vegetables stand for a few minutes after chopping as this creates many healthy compounds.

CABBAGE AND APPLE SALAD

175g/6oz red cabbage, shredded
175g/6oz green cabbage, shredded
2 tbsp olive oil
1 tbsp lemon juice
1 clove garlic, crushed
4 apples, chopped

Mix together the shredded cabbages, olive oil, lemon juice and garlic in a large bowl. Refrigerate for at least 2 hours until ready to serve. Add the apple, season if desired and serve immediately.

◎ ✋ ♥ Ⓒ

leek

The benefits of the life-extending allium family with a milder taste.

Being a member of the same family as onions and garlic, the leek shares many of those vegetables' life-saving qualities. Eaten regularly, they help to bring blood pressure down to healthy levels. They also reduce the risk of strokes and heart disease by combating harmful LDL cholesterol and increasing levels of the 'good' cholesterol, HDL. This helps to keep the arteries clear and supple by preventing a build-up of plaque. They also combat prostate and colon cancer, both reducing the risk and slowing the growth of tumours. Leeks contain less of the protective compounds than onions or garlic, but their milder taste allows them to be eaten in larger amounts.

NUTRIENTS
Vitamins B6, C, folic acid; iron, manganese; fibre

Lightly steamed leeks are perfect to offset the oiliness of omega-3-rich fish.

LEEK AND POTATO SOUP

3 tbsp olive oil
2 cloves garlic, crushed
2 potatoes, peeled and grated
450g/1lb leeks, sliced
1 litre/35fl oz/4 cups stock
pepper to taste
2 tbsp chopped parsley

Heat the oil in a frying pan and fry the garlic for 1 minute. Add the potatoes and leeks and sauté for 5–10 minutes. Add the stock and bring to the boil. Reduce the heat and simmer for 30 minutes. Blend if required. Stir in pepper, garnish with parsley and serve.

lettuce

Add a lettuce leaf to that sandwich and divide your risk of a hip fracture in half.

NUTRIENTS
Vitamins B1, B2, C, K, beta-carotene, folic acid; chromium, iron, manganese, molybdenum, phosphorus, potassium; fibre

It looks insubstantial, but a lettuce leaf could be a powerful protector against one of the most frequent accidents that disable older people. Scientists have found that older women who eat lettuce every day have half as many hip fractures as those who eat it less than once a week. It's the vitamin K content that does so much good. Any kind of lettuce helps, but, as with other leafy foods, the darker colour is a sign of more nutritional value.

The dark green leaves of the cos, or romaine, are the most nutrient-rich of all lettuces.

PEAS AND LETTUCE

55g/2oz butter
350g/12oz peas
8 large cos lettuce leaves, cut into strips
4 tbsp stock or water
1 tsp pepper

Melt the butter over a gentle heat and add the peas and lettuce. Add the stock or water and bring to the boil, then simmer, covered, for 5 minutes. Season with pepper and serve.

mushroom

All kinds of mushrooms are now known to combat cancer and age-related diseases.

Mushrooms are one of the richest sources of a powerful antioxidant called L-ergothioneine, which combats cell damage. They are also rich in vitamin B3, which may slow the onset of age-related dementias, and potassium, which helps to regulate blood pressure. Research is being done into their cancer-fighting properties, including reducing the risk of breast cancer. And their minerals may ease the pain of arthritis. Mushrooms may also help to slow down age-related muscle loss, as they provide protein in a form that the body can easily use. Shiitake mushrooms, in particular, are rich in iron.

NUTRIENTS
Vitamin B-complex, biotin, folic acid; copper, manganese, phosphorus, potassium, selenium, zinc; protein; tryptophan

BLACK AND WHITE MUSHROOMS

½ tbsp olive oil
8 large portobello mushrooms
4 slices wholemeal bread
55g/2oz halloumi cheese
1 tbsp soy sauce

Place the mushrooms face-down on a grill and brush lightly with oil. Grill for 3 minutes until tender. Repeat on the other side. Meanwhile, toast the bread in a toaster. Top 4 of the mushrooms with halloumi cheese and grill for 2 minutes. Pour soy sauce onto the remaining mushrooms. Serve on the toast.

olive

Snack on olives to keep your skin youthful, while oiling your joints and protecting your cells.

Olives, and their extra-virgin oil, are among the best sources of monounsaturated fats. They are also rich in vitamin E and polyphenols. These three nutrients are associated with a lower risk of colon cancer, which becomes increasingly common in later age. Together, these nutrients protect cells from the damage that can lead to cancer, as well as causing heart disease, hardening of the arteries and skin deterioration. Their soothing effects on tissue may ease the pain of arthritis. The vitamin E content can reduce the severity of hot flushes.

NUTRIENTS
Vitamin E; calcium, copper, iron; polyphenols; fibre

TAPENADE

200g/7oz olives, pitted and chopped
55g/2oz capers, drained and chopped
55g/2oz anchovies, chopped (optional)
juice of 1 lemon
1 tsp ground black pepper
2 tsp olive oil

Place all the ingredients in a bowl. Mix well, or briefly blend in a blender for a smooth texture. Serve on fresh bread or as a dip with crudités.

silver beet

This leafy life-enhancer adds a beauty secret to its health-protective qualities.

Silver beet, or Swiss chard, is one of those leafy dark green superveg that counteracts many of the ills of middle and later age, including various cancers. It contains an unusually high number of vitamins and minerals. Among their many other benefits, magnesium and vitamin K keep bones strong; potassium protects the heart; beta carotene prevents DNA damage; and vitamin E keeps skin young, while reducing the risk of Alzheimer's. And they all work together to be health-protective.

NUTRIENTS

Vitamins A, B-complex, C, E, K; calcium, copper, iron, magnesium, manganese, phosphorus, potassium, zinc; fibre; protein

SILVER BEET AU GRATIN

450g/1lb silver beet
1 tbsp olive oil
4 cloves garlic, crushed
400g/14oz tin tomatoes
115g/4oz cheese, grated
2 tsp lemon juice

Strip the leaves from the beet and chop. Slice the stems, boil for 10 minutes and drain. Heat the oil and sauté the garlic for 1 minute. Add the tomatoes and cook for 5 minutes. Pour over the stems in a baking dish. Top with the cheese and grill for 3–5 minutes. Steam the leaves, add lemon juice and serve with the gratin.

squash

This bright orange superveg gives a boost to the body's cellular defences.

NUTRIENTS
Vitamins B1, B3, B5, B6, C, beta carotene, folic acid; copper, manganese, potassium; fibre; omega-3 oils

The solid flesh of squashes, such as butternut and pumpkin, provides a healthy dose of age-defying nutrients. Extracts from squash have been found to help ease benign prostatic hypertrophy, which bedevils many older men as the prostate gland becomes enlarged. Regularly eating squash may help to prevent it developing. Their rich array of nutrients, including beta-cryptoxanthin, counteract the cell damage that leads to cancer and heart disease. And they have anti-inflammatory properties that could relieve the pain of many age-related conditions.

ROAST BUTTERNUT SQUASH WITH CHEESE AND WALNUTS

4 tbsp olive oil
2 cloves garlic, crushed
2 butternut squash, halved and deseeded
200g/7oz cheese, cubed
100g/3½ oz/1 cup walnut halves

Preheat the oven to 190°C/375°F/ Gas 5. Place the olive oil and garlic in the hollow of each squash. Roast the squash for an hour, until tender. Scoop out most of the flesh, leaving enough to keep the shape. Mix together the flesh with the cheese and walnuts. Place in skins, cook for a few minutes until the cheese is soft, and serve immediately.

oregano

One of the best antioxidants in the kitchen, this leafy herb helps prevent cancer and heart disease.

Herbs and fruits are among the best providers of antioxidants – nutrients that help protect the body's cells from damage caused as a side effect of natural processes. But when researchers tested dozens of different plants, they found that oregano offers four times more protection than even that antioxidant celebrity, the blueberry. Its antioxidant qualities combat the conditions of ageing, especially heart disease and cancers. Oregano is also known for its antibacterial qualities, which may offer protection against food-borne diseases, which are more dangerous to older people. Freshly picked leaves are the most effective.

NUTRIENTS
Vitamins C, K, beta carotene; calcium, iron, magnesium, manganese; omega-3 oils

One tablespoon of oregano leaves provides as much antioxidant as a whole apple.

SCRAMBLE MED

1 tbsp olive oil
2 cloves garlic, crushed
200g/7oz spinach
8 eggs, beaten
200g/7oz feta cheese (optional)
4 tbsp torn oregano leaves

Heat the oil over a low heat and sauté the garlic for 30 seconds.

Add the spinach and cook for 2 minutes. Beat together 3 tablespoons of water and the eggs and pour over the spinach. Stir continuously so the eggs cook evenly. Crumble in the feta, if using, for the final minute of cooking time. Stir in the oregano and serve immediately.

oats

NUTRIENTS
Vitamin B1; magnesium, manganese, phosphorus, selenium; fibre; protein

OAT CAKES

100g/3½oz/¾ cup fine oatmeal
pinch of bicarbonate of soda
pinch of salt
1 tbsp olive oil

Preheat the oven to 180°C/350°F/Gas 4. Mix together the oatmeal, bicarbonate of soda and salt. Add the oil and 2 tablespoons of hot water and mix well until a firm dough. Roll out on a floured surface. Cut into 8 rounds, place on a greased baking tray and bake for 8–10 minutes until browned. Serve.

A bowl of porridge for breakfast could turn out to be the healthiest meal of the day.

Could something as simple as oats provide an answer to heart disease, diabetes and strokes? Eaten regularly, all kinds of whole grains are associated with good health in older people, but oats have special qualities. They contain a form of fibre called beta-glucan, which has an exceptional ability to reduce cholesterol – cutting the risk of strokes and heart disease from blocked arteries – and to stabilize blood sugar. Other compounds in oats protect the heart and lungs, reduce the risk of cancer and even increase the body's ability to fight off infectious diseases.

salmon

Oily fish counteract dryness and stiffness by lubricating the joints, eyes and arteries.

Salmon is an excellent source of omega-3 fatty acids, which counteract many of the effects of ageing. By preserving brain and cell functions, they protect against numerous diseases including cancers, age-related eye disease, strokes, forgetfulness and dementia. They also fight heart disease by lowering cholesterol and other blood lipids, preventing arrhythmia, reducing blood pressure and making blood less likely to clot. Their powerful anti-inflammatory effects ease the pain and stiffness of arthritis.

NUTRIENTS
Vitamins B3, B6, B12; magnesium, phosphorus, selenium; protein; tryptophan

SALMON IN GRAPE SAUCE

2 tsp mustard
2 tsp dried thyme
2 tsp honey
4 salmon fillets
1 tbsp olive oil
225g/8oz red grapes, halved
125ml/4fl oz/½ cup red wine

Preheat the oven to 150°C/ 300°F/Gas 2. Mix together the mustard, thyme and honey and rub into the fish. Heat half the oil in a pan and brown both sides of the salmon. Transfer to an oiled baking tray and bake for 10 minutes. Heat the remaining oil in a pan and sauté the grapes for 2 minutes, add the wine, bring to the boil and reduce by half. Pour over the salmon and serve.

walnut

This powerful snack protects the heart, boosts brain power and even helps you sleep well.

NUTRIENTS
Copper, manganese; omega-3 oils; tryptophan

NUTRIENTS
Copper, manganese; omega-3 oils; tryptophan

Walnuts have also been found to reduce the risk of developing gallstones.

SPICY WALNUTS

1 tbsp curry paste
1 tsp mango juice
1 tsp cumin
115g/4oz/1 cup walnuts

Preheat the oven to 180°C/ 350°F/Gas 4. Mix together the curry paste, mango juice and cumin into a smooth paste. Coat the walnuts and place on an oiled baking tray and cook for 5–10 minutes until crisp. Serve as a snack.

Eating walnuts at the end of a rich meal can counter the effects of the fat you've eaten by reducing inflammation and keeping the arteries flexible, scientists have found. Walnuts are one of the richest sources of antioxidants. They protect the heart in numerous ways, preventing arrhythmia as well as lowering cholesterol and protecting the arteries.

One of walnut's most valuable effects is in fighting inflammation. This means a lot more than just relieving sore skin and painful joints, especially as you grow older. Inflammation plays a role in many of the most debilitating conditions of age. It hardens the arteries, causing high blood pressure, strokes and heart disease. It speeds up thinning of the bones, leading to osteoporosis. The damage caused by chronic inflammation has been linked with the development of cancers. And it is implicated in degenerative diseases of both brain and body. Eating just half a dozen walnuts a day is enough to reduce your risk.

Friendly fats

Eating nuts may reduce the risk of developing diabetes, but if you already have it, walnuts provide the right balance of fats in your diet. Unlike most nuts, they are rich in polyunsaturated fat. They are also among the best sources of alpha-linolenic acid, a form of omega-3 fatty acid. Omega-3 helps keep cells strong and flexible, protecting against the illnesses of ageing and keeping the brain in top condition. If all that's not enough to give you good dreams, walnuts promote healthy sleep by regulating the body's melatonin production.

WALNUT AND BANANA WHIRL

2 ripe bananas, chopped
250ml/9fl oz/1 cup low-fat yogurt
8 tbsp walnuts, chopped
2 tbsp honey

Place the bananas in a blender. Add the yogurt, half the walnuts and the honey. Blend, on a low speed at first, until smooth. Serve immediately, topped with the remaining walnuts.

red wine

NUTRIENTS
Vitamins B1, B6, C, E; manganese, potassium; flavonoids; polyphenols

The health-protective powers of this drink aren't just down to the relaxing effects of alcohol.

Red wine is a central element of the Mediterranean diet, which is credited with promoting long life and low rates of heart disease. Its nutrients reduce cholesterol and blood pressure, keep heart muscles supple and prevent blood clots. One of these is resveratrol, which

> The wine-making process makes some of the nutrients easier for the body to use.

may also protect the body's cells from cancerous changes. And a glass a day has been found to reduce the risk of Alzheimer's, by preventing plaque building up in the brain. But drinking more than a unit a day (women) or two (men) reduces these benefits, which at larger levels are outweighed by alcohol damage.

MULLED WINE

750ml/26fl oz bottle red wine
1 orange, scrubbed and halved
2 tbsp honey
2.5cm/1in root ginger, finely chopped
1 tsp cinnamon

Put all the ingredients in a saucepan. Bring to just below the boil and simmer for 20 minutes, stirring occasionally. Ladle into cups and serve.

tea

Take a tea break: the 200 active compounds in an everyday cuppa are working while you relax.

Ordinary tea has been found to have an extraordinary number of health-protective qualities. Tea is, surprisingly, a very rich source of the plant compounds called flavonoids that protect the heart. Only apples, onions and broccoli equal tea's ability to reduce the risk of heart disease by 20 per cent. And for those who are already affected, just one or two cups a day may halve the risk of a second heart attack. Tea has antibacterial qualities and may combat cancers of the digestive system. It reduces the effects of stress, increases mental alertness and may help to protect bones from osteoporosis.

NUTRIENTS
Vitamins B1, B2, B6, C, K, beta carotene, folic acid; fluorine, manganese, potassium, zinc; flavonoids

BARA BRITH: WELSH TEA BREAD

350g/12oz/2¾ cups dried fruit
375ml/13fl oz/1½ cups black tea
200g/7oz/1 cup brown sugar
600g/1lb 5oz/4¾ cups self-raising flour
1 tsp cinnamon
1 egg, beaten

Soak the fruit overnight in the tea. The following day, preheat the oven to 160°C/325°F/Gas 3. Mix together the sugar, flour and cinnamon with the fruit. Add the egg and mix well. Bake in a greased 2lb loaf tin for 1½ hours. Leave to cool, then slice, spread with butter and serve.

ailments directory

ANAEMIA

The first sign that you're short of red blood cells is usually weakness or exhaustion. The likeliest cause is lack of iron or vitamin B12. Young women, in particular, are at risk, especially if they have heavy periods and eat little or no meat, as the body absorbs iron more easily from meat or fish than from any other source. Foods rich in vitamin C help the body absorb iron. If the exhaustion continues, see your doctor.

Try more:

chickpeas, mussels, venison, prunes, green beans, spinach, yogurt, eggs, sea vegetables, sweet potatoes, oysters, milk, salmon

ARTHRITIS

Osteoarthritis is caused by wear and tear on the joints, so most people have at least a few twinges by the time they reach their 50s. It may also happen earlier at the site of an injury. The degenerative disease rheumatoid arthritis is much less common but often starts in younger people. They're different conditions, but both may respond to the anti-inflammatory effects of foods rich in omega-3, especially oily fish (though oily fish is not recommended for anyone with the form of arthritis called gout). Calcium, iron and vitamin D have shown some good effects on arthritis. A diet rich in fruit and vegetables provides many other phytonutrients that are believed to be helpful.

Try more:

turmeric, curly endive, ginger, pineapples, green beans, cherries, pomegranates, aubergines, cabbage, mushrooms, olive oil, squash, salmon

ASTHMA AND LUNG DISEASE

Foods rich in vitamin C have long been known to fight asthma and other chest diseases. Other nutrients are now known to help in different ways: magnesium, for example, helps prevent the breath-restricting spasms of an asthma attack.

Try more:

kiwi fruit, oranges, kale, onions, red peppers, mustard, mussels, rosemary, olive oil

CANCERS

Healthy eating could prevent up to a third of all cancers, according to the World Health Organization. There are a huge number of naturally occurring phytonutrients shown to reduce cancer risk. Fruits and vegetables of every kind offer slightly different beneficial compounds.

Try more:

oranges, raspberries, carrots, kale, onions, red peppers, turmeric, mussels, venison, apples, beetroot, broccoli, cauliflower, cumin, ginger, watercress, grapefruit, pears, rock melon, strawberries, garlic,

rye, brown rice, blueberries, cherries, pomegranate, aubergine, cabbage, leeks, mushrooms, olives, silver beet, squash, oregano, oats, salmon, red wine

CYSTITIS

Urinary tract infections such as cystitis cause intense pain and difficulty in passing urine. They must always be treated, as they can spread fast and affect the kidneys. Vitamin C combats infection, and some foods have been found to discourage bacteria from sticking to the bladder wall. These foods are a back-up to treatment, and they reduce the risk of recurrence.

Try more:

cranberries, alfalfa sprouts, blueberries, cherries

DEPRESSION

The body converts nutrients into message-carrying chemicals that have a direct effect on our emotions. Nutrient deficiencies can cause psychological problems in vulnerable people. People who are feeling down often neglect themselves, so the condition is exacerbated by poor diet. Cheer yourself up with foods rich in tryptophan, selenium, B vitamins and protein.

Try more:

apricots, bananas, avocados, sea vegetables, sweet potatoes, brown rice, Brazil nuts, linseed, oysters, milk

DIABETES

Foods that release glucose slowly into the bloodstream help to keep diabetes under control, and may also reduce the risk of developing this disease. Avoid processed foods and, although dried fruit and juices are healthy foods, limit these too as they are rich in sugars.

Try more:

oranges, grapefruit, garlic, almond, tofu, green tea, sweet potato, cinnamon, oats, walnuts

ENERGY AND MOOD SWINGS

Fluctuating blood-sugar levels can cause mood swings and make you hyperactive one moment, tired and stressed the next. This is usually caused by highly processed or sugary foods and can lead to other health problems, including diabetes. Aim for foods that have a gently regulating effect on blood sugar.

Try more:

oranges, raspberries, kale, chickpeas, honey, prunes, black beans, lentils, grapefruit, courgettes, peas, rye, tofu, green tea, sweet potatoes, cinnamon, brown rice, blueberries, leeks, oats, walnuts

FATIGUE

If you're getting seven to eight hours' sleep a night but feel exhausted most of the time, you may not be eating all the many nutrients you need, including protein, B vitamins and an array of minerals. This often happens when you're busy, too, and living on fast food. Or you may be suffering from borderline anaemia or depression. You probably need to improve your diet generally. Unexplained fatigue can be a sign of something more serious, so if cutting down on stress, working sensible hours and eating well doesn't help, seek medical advice.

Try more:

wheat germ, cashews, tuna, bananas, asparagus, Brazil nuts, sunflower seeds, mushrooms

HEADACHES AND MIGRAINE

These can be triggered by a number of different stimuli, from tiredness to expansion of blood vessels in the head. They may be prevented, or relieved, by foods rich in omega-3 oils, vitamin B2, magnesium or calcium. Some migraines can be triggered by eating preserved meat, strong cheeses, pickles, fatty foods, coffee or the artificial sweetener aspartame.

Try more:

chickpeas, venison, cottage cheese, sea vegetables, milk

HEART DISEASE

Healthy eating is proven to play a major role in preventing or alleviating heart disease. All kinds of fruit and vegetables are especially valuable, particularly when they are replacing high-fat foods or heavily processed items that are low in nutritional value.

Try more:

kiwi fruit, onions, mussels, apples, broccoli, grapes, green beans, pumpkin seeds, cashew nuts, grapefruit, garlic, tofu, green tea, apricots, brown rice, blueberries, cherries, pomegranates, aubergines, leeks, olive oil, silver beet, squash, oregano, oats, salmon, walnuts, red wine, tea

HIGH BLOOD PRESSURE

Hypertension, or high blood pressure, increases the risk of heart disease and strokes. Exercise and stress-reduction can bring it down, as can losing excess weight. Avoid high-fat dishes and salty foods.

Try more:

apples, celery, potatoes, spinach, garlic, avocado, sea vegetables, figs, pomegranate, leeks, mushrooms, salmon, red wine

INFECTIONS

Viral and bacterial infections usually attack the respiratory or digestive systems. Foods rich in vitamin C strengthen the body's defences against infections, and some foods contain specific antibacterial compounds. Drinks made with cider vinegar or fresh lemon

juice and honey can ease the common throat and head symptoms.

Try more:

cranberries, kiwi fruit, oranges, raspberries, Brussels sprouts, kale, onions, red peppers, basil, cloves, coriander, chickpeas, honey, lemons, broccoli, cumin, ginger, peppermint, yogurt, garlic, chillies, aubergines, oats, oregano, tea

IRRITABLE BOWEL SYNDROME (IBS)

This distressing and sometimes painful condition can involve constipation, diarrhoea, flatulence, nausea or all of these. Bouts may be triggered by stress or by certain foods such as dairy products, spicy foods or the artificial sweetener sorbitol.

Tea, coffee and alcohol can also have an irritating effect. As IBS sometimes develops from chronic constipation, it may be relieved by the same remedies: fibre-rich foods, some exercise every day, plenty of fluids, regular meals not too late in the evening, unhurried bowel movements. If flatulence is a problem, don't eat a lot of pulses.

Try more:
raspberries, apples, artichoke, cucumber, black pepper, cumin, ginger, peppermint, pears, figs, prunes

MEMORY LOSS
Forgetfulness, inability to concentrate and 'brain fog' can stem from many causes, often including stress and tiredness. Some nutrients are known to help keep your brain sharp at any age, including omega-3 oils and compounds in certain herbs. These may also delay or prevent mental deterioration in later life.

Try more:
sea vegetables, cinnamon, rosemary, sage, kidney beans, sunflower seeds, linseed, oysters, milk, blueberries, salmon, tea

MENOPAUSAL SYMPTOMS
Levels of the reproductive hormone oestrogen can rise and fall sharply during the few years leading up to the menopause, and then decline steeply afterwards. This sometimes causes disruptive symptoms, which can be alleviated through healthy eating. Phytoestrogens help to replace some of the missing oestrogen. Foods rich in vitamin E can reduce the severity of hot flushes and prevent night sweats causing insomnia. Depression, fatigue and memory loss may also occur during this time.

Try more:
rye, tofu, sea vegetables, sage, brown rice, sunflower seeds, linseed, olive oil, silver beet

OSTEOPOROSIS
Building strong bones before your 30s reduces the risk that you'll suffer from this brittle-bone condition in later life. Weight-bearing exercise is vital, and getting out in the sunshine lets your body produce vitamin D, which helps turn the calcium you eat into bone. Dairy foods and oily fish also provide vitamin D.

Vitamin K and several other minerals are also important. All of these can also delay the progression of osteoporosis if you already have it.

Try more:

kale, onions, green beans, spinach, cashew nuts, chicken, cheese, peas, rocket, soy, sea vegetables, figs, cherries, lettuce, olive oil, silver beet, tea

PREMENSTRUAL SYNDROME (PMS)

If you feel depressed or irritable, especially during the couple of days before a period, but fine once it starts, you probably have PMS. Sugary or fatty comfort foods can make the symptoms worse, but foods rich in vitamins B6, D and E, magnesium and calcium can help a lot.

Try more:

cottage cheese, banana, sweet potato, linseed, milk

STOMACH ULCERS

These painful patches of damage to the stomach wall are now known to be caused by the bacterium *Helicobacter pylori*, and can often be cured by antibiotics. Ulcers can be exacerbated by stress or erratic eating habits. Some powerful antibacterial foods can reduce the risk of developing them.

Try more:

oranges, broccoli, yogurt, garlic, chillies, bananas

STRESS

The right foods can calm anxiety and irritation just as they can lift depression. Pulses, for example, contain plenty of potassium for calmness and magnesium to promote relaxation.

Try more:

bananas, asparagus, avocado, sea vegetables, kidney beans, brown rice, Brazil nuts, sunflower seeds, linseed, tea

THRUSH

This itchy yeast infection most commonly affects the genitals. The discomfort can be eased by daubing with yogurt or bathing with diluted cider vinegar. Wearing loose cotton clothes and avoiding hot baths can also help. Some foods discourage the growth of yeasts, which cause fungal infections.

Try more:

raspberries, yogurt, alfalfa sprouts, cinnamon

glossary

Anthocyanin A flavonoid that gives plants a blue to purple colour and has strong health-protective effects.

Antioxidant A substance, naturally occurring in many plants, believed to protect cells from damage from free radicals.

Bacteria Microscopic single-celled organisms, some of which aid bodily functions while others can cause disease.

Beta carotene A nutrient found in fruit and vegetables, which the body turns into vitamin A.

Blood sugar, or blood glucose The form in which fuel from food is carried in the blood to provide energy to cells. A diet of highly processed foods may make blood-sugar levels fluctuate unhealthily, causing mood swings and energy slumps. The body produces a hormone called insulin to prevent blood-sugar levels rising excessively. In diabetes, the body is no longer able to produce enough insulin to regulate blood-sugar levels effectively.

Carbohydrates Starchy or sweet foods that provide energy. The body breaks them down into glucose, for immediate fuel, and glycogen, which is stored in the liver and muscles for future use.

Carcinogen Anything that can cause cancer.

Carotenoids Antioxidants, found mainly in vegetables, that have been shown to reduce the risk of many diseases (including cancers) and enhance the immune system.

Cholesterol A fatty substance made (from dietary fat) in the body and needed for purposes such as building cell walls. If too much is produced, it can line artery walls, restricting the flow of blood to the heart and brain. Low-density lipoprotein (LDL), or 'bad cholesterol', increases the risk of this, whereas high-density lipoprotein (HDL) or 'good cholesterol' helps remove fats from the bloodstream.

Cruciferous vegetables An exceptionally beneficial plant family including cauliflower,

Brussels sprouts and numerous dark-green leafy vegetables.

Detoxification The body's natural process of eliminating toxic substances, which can be promoted by eating certain foods.

Diuretic Something that encourages increased urination.

Enzyme A protein that facilitates the body's chemical reactions, such as digestion.

Fat One of three necessary food groups (along with carbohydrates and protein), fat is used for numerous purposes including cell maintenance and absorption of certain vitamins. Monounsaturated and polyunsaturated fats are considered healthiest. An excess of saturated fat, mainly from animal products, can cause high blood-cholesterol levels. Hydrogenated fat, found mainly in processed foods, is now considered harmful to health.

Fibre Plant matter that the body does not absorb but that aids the process of digestion. Soluble fibre is thought to help control blood sugar and cholesterol. Insoluble fibre aids elimination.

Flavonoids Plant compounds that seem to strengthen the body's ability to resist cell damage, inflammation and infection.

Free radical An unstable molecule (formed as a by-product of the body's natural functions) that may damage cells, leading to diseases such as cancer.

Glycaemic index (GI) A measure of how quickly the body turns foods into glucose. Low-GI foods are healthier as they release glucose slowly, helping to control blood-sugar levels and appetite.

Glycogen The form in which energy is stored in the muscles for later use.

HDL See cholesterol.

Hydrochloric acid The main component of the acids that digest food in the stomach.

Hypertension High blood pressure, sometimes caused by a build-up of plaque in the arteries.

LDL See cholesterol.

Leptin A hormone that controls the appetite; it may be stimulated by omega-3 oils.

Lignans Antioxidant chemicals found in certain plants that, being similar in structure to the hormone oestrogen, may relieve menopausal symptoms.

Lycopene A powerful carotenoid found in red fruit and vegetables.

Nitrates Food preservatives that have been linked with cancer.

Omega-3 oils (or fats, or fatty acids). A group of polyunsaturated fats, mainly found in oily fish, believed to provide many health benefits to mind and body.

Oxalates Substances occurring naturally in certain foods that, in susceptible people, can damage the gall bladder or kidneys.

Perimenopause The time leading up to and just after a woman's final menstrual period.

Phytonutrients Beneficial compounds found in plants.

Phytosterol Substances which are found in plants that may lower cholesterol levels.

Plaque One form, made from cholesterol and other fats, builds up on the lining of arteries and can restrict blood flow. Another form is made from protein fragments that clump together in the brain and is linked with Alzheimer's disease.

Polyphenol A form of antioxidant chemical.

Protein An essential food group, needed for the growth and repair of tissue. Most abundant in foods of animal origin, but nuts, seeds and pulses are also good sources.

Pulses Dried beans, the large seeds of several members of the Fabaceae family. Examples in this book are black beans, kidney beans, chickpeas, soy beans (in the form of tofu) and lentils.

Resveratrol A cancer-fighting compound found in several plants, including red or blue berries and grapes (and therefore red wine).

Serotonin A chemical produced by nerve cells that lifts the mood; also found in some foods.

Tryptophan An amino acid that the brain converts into the 'feel-good' chemical serotonin.

index